HOME HEALTH OUTCOMES

PAY *for* PERFORMANCE

DISEASE MANAGEMENT

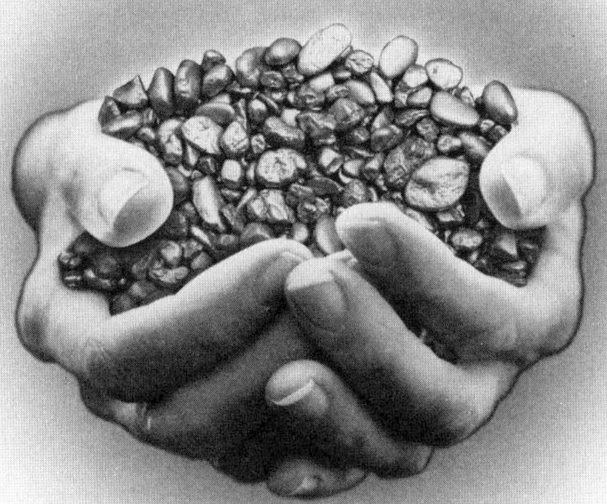

Gold Nuggets for Success!

Melinda H. Huffman, BSN, MSN, CCNS
Principal
Disease Management/Outcomes Specialist
Miller & Huffman Outcome Architects, LLC

Published by Miller & Huffman Outcome Architects, LLC
Winchester, Tennessee USA
www.outcome-architects.com

This publication is sold directly by Miller & Huffman Outcome Architects, LLC and through authorized resellers.
For orders and information, contact:
Miller & Huffman Outcome Architects, LLC
269 Lakeview Way
Winchester, TN 37398
Phone/Fax: 931.967.0894
Email: info@outcome-architects.com
www.outcome-architects.com

Cover Design and Interior Layout:
Stephen Hefner, Brunswick, GA

Printing: RJ Communications, LLC
New York, New York, USA

Disclaimer
Strategies and methods in this book are compilations of the author's research of the literature and Miller & Huffman Outcome Architects, LLC experience and expertise. Because the information contained herein may be used in a myriad of ways, the author and Miller & Huffman Outcome Architects, LLC disclaim any specific result for the user.

ISBN-13: 978-0-9793131-0-3
ISBN-10: 0-9793131-0-4

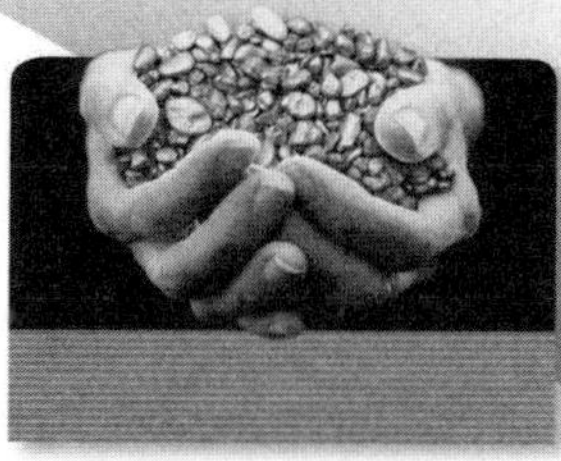

Table of Contents

Table of Contents

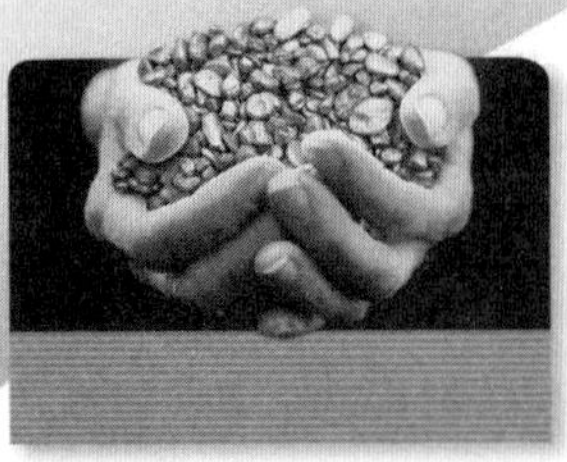

Introduction

Introduction

Healthcare providers have their ears to the ground for information on how to succeed in an outcomes-driven pay-for-performance environment. Vendors and suppliers want to know how best to serve and support the home health market. The principals of *Miller & Huffman Outcome Architects, LLC* have researched hundreds of resources and share methods from years of success in outcomes management to bring the user drill-down, have-to-know information to better manage home health outcomes, reduce acute care hospitalization, implement successful disease management programs, enhance marketing efforts, increase market share and thrive in pay-for-performance.

This resource is designed to provide step-by-step guidance, to save time, and to allow the user to customize these strategies to his/her organization. Because there are many resources available for learning OASIS and OBQI, this resource does not include an in-depth reiteration of these processes or procedures.

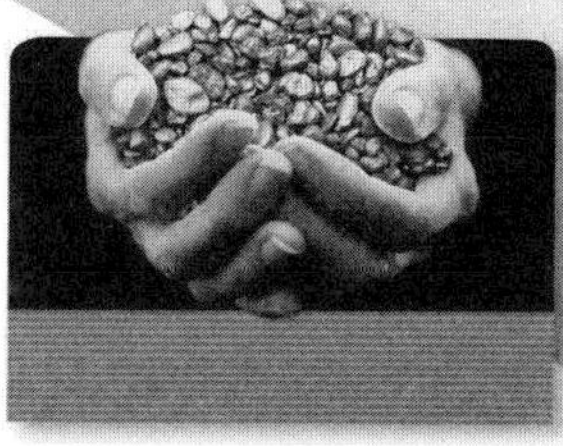

Guidelines for Use

This book is a compilation of proven strategies and methods in helping home health providers, hospitals, outpatient clinics, and product vendors improve outcomes of home health quality, disease management, finance, and marketing, all key ingredients in succeeding in an outcomes-driven, pay-for-performance environment.

These methods are designed in a step-by-step format to educate and offer guidance to:

- Home health quality managers
- Executives, agency directors and managers
- Staff development and performance improvement coordinators
- Home health staff
- New home health employees
- Hospital administrators and staff
- Suppliers and vendors
- Payers
- Other healthcare professionals
- Organizations who desire to know more about partnering with and/or servicing the home health provider

Gold Nuggets for Success can be used to:

- Orient new employees
- Educate staff
- Plan business strategy
- Plan performance improvement activities
- Develop a disease management action plan
- Improve outcomes
- Enhance profitability
- Implement new marketing strategies
- Determine technology needs
- Enhance collaboration with referral sources
- Achieve wound care quality and profitability
- Prepare for pay-for-performance

This resource contains five primary sections.

Section 1 serves as a *Pay for Performance Primer*. It outlines P4P principles, describes what it is and its purpose, summarizes the P4P home health demonstration project, and discusses the goals of CMS related to P4P. It gives the quality measures for home health, physicians, hospitals, and nursing homes to assist users in collaborating across healthcare settings to improve care quality, efficiency, and to reduce costs across the continuum.

Section 2 contains step-by-step *Solutions for Success* to help agencies succeed in home health outcomes-driven pay-for-performance. These solutions have direct application to home health outcomes management.

Section 3 gives *Terms, Definitions and Examples* used frequently in home health. It is divided into three subsections.

Subsection A contains general terms related to home health, disease management, outcomes and managed care.

Subsection B contains technology terms.

Subsection C contains sales and marketing terms.

The term(s) are listed alphabetically in categories that are identified by each letter of the alphabet. For example, the term Adverse Event is listed alphabetically in category "A". The term, Benchmark is listed alphabetically in category "B", and so on. Terms follow in alphabetical order within each subsequent alphabetical "letter" category. The definition is followed by a home health example, as needed.

Section 4 contains a list of *Acronyms* (and websites if applicable) commonly used in home health. This list was compiled by the author and verified with the listing of acronyms for all healthcare settings provided by the Center for Medicare and Medicaid Services. The complete CMS acronym listing may be found at: www.cms.hhs.gov/apps/acronyms/listall.asp/

Section 5 contains a listing of *Websites for Evidence-Based Practice* that agencies can access for managing patients with chronic conditions most often cared for in the home health setting.

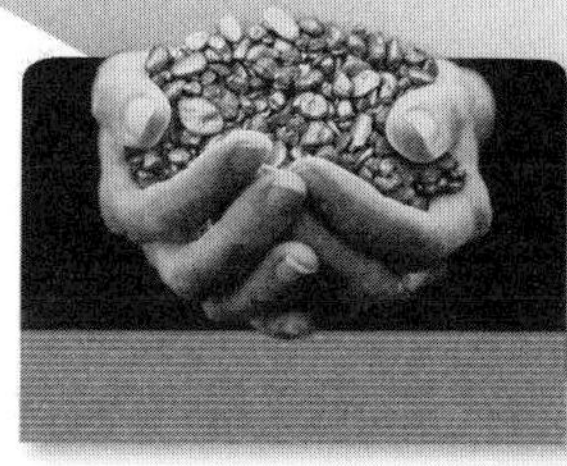

Acknowledgements

Untold appreciation to Colleen Miller whose vast experience and expertise in DM clinical and financial outcomes management is reflected in many of the outcome-based solutions and strategies contained herein. As the partner in Miller & Huffman Outcome Architects, LLC, her commitment to excellence is unending and her ability unmatched.

Special thanks to Laurie Salmons with 20 years of healthcare sales experience, who contributed to the terms and definitions for sales and marketing.

Grateful acknowledgement of Ty Bello, President of Team at Work, Fort Wayne, IN, an accomplished, certified business coach and HME specialist, who collaborated with me on health and business coaching, and who contributed the nugget on distributor alliances.

Sincere gratitude to Betty Deblasio of QSource, the Quality Improvement Organization of Tennessee, whose many years of home health experience and expertise were critical.

Many thanks to Keri Ruffell of SHP, Strategic Healthcare Programs, of Santa Barbara, California, whose vast experience in sales and marketing of technology tremendously enhanced the meaningfulness and usfulness of this resource.

Special appreciation to Mary McGoldrick of Home Health Systems, Inc. for sharing her immense content expertise and guidance.

Immense gratitude to my friend Stephen Hefner, whose talent in graphic design and content layout is simply unsurpassed.

Melinda H. Huffman

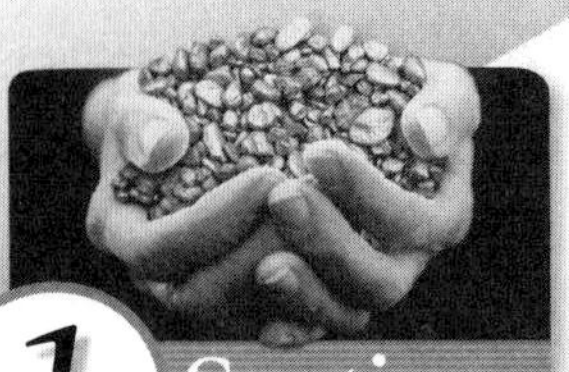

1 Section

Pay for Performance Primer

» What is pay-for-performance (P4P)?

Pay-for-performance is a budget neutral approach to enhance healthcare quality and efficiency by giving providers financial incentives for improved clinical outcomes, cost containment and patient satisfaction (Baker, 2003). Pay-for-performance, also known as quality based purchasing, ties a portion of reimbursement to delivery of care that has been proven to be effective (USDHHS, "Overview. Home").

» Why P4P?

Pay-for-performance evolved in response to:

- Rising healthcare costs, increased utilization
- Increase in the number of persons with chronic conditions
- Demand for consumer-directed care
- Demand for improvement in the quality of care (Baker, 2003)
- Medical error rate more frequent and harmful than previously thought (Institute of Medicine, 2001)

» Goals of CMS Driving P4P

(Remington, 2006)

1. Facilitate collaboration across healthcare settings
2. Reduce clinical practice variation through use of evidence-based practice interventions
3. Reduce unplanned hospitalizations
4. Reduce emergency care use
5. Improve care efficiency
6. Reduce healthcare spending

CMS Premise for Improving Quality Outcomes and Reducing Costs:

- Collaboration among stakeholders
- Effective coordination of chronic illness care
- Program development and partnerships
- Disease management/outcome specialists to support providers

Emerging CMS Priorities for Healthcare

While the current home health assessment and reporting tool, OASIS, will remain in use in the forseeable future, several new priorities have emerged and are expected to be part of planning for the future:

- Pay-for-performance – tying a portion of reimbursement to delivery of care that has been proven to be effective
- Standardizing assessment/quality measurement across post-acute health care settings
- Integration of measures of process and systems
- Electronic Health Record (EHR)

It is too early to know what forms these priorities may take. Pay-for-performance logically will link to actual activities and efforts of providers using evidence-based practices and systems (in the form of structural measures that will be collected at the agency level) to promote use of such practices. Planning/discussions are in a preliminary phase. Providers, consumers, and interested parties, such as the many organizations that represent and work with patients in post-acute, home, community, and long-term care settings, will be part of these efforts as they evolve (USDHHS, 2006, May).

» What are the Draft P4P Timeline & Incentives?

2007: Home health agencies that submit the required quality data using the Outcome Assessment and Information Set (OASIS) will receive payments based on the full home health market basket update for calendar year (CY) 2007. If a home health agency does not submit quality data, the home health market basket will be reduced by 2 percentage points for CY 2007.

In accordance with the Deficit Reduction Act (DRA), the Home Health Agency Preview Reports will be made available to home health agencies on an annual basis. The reports will be placed in a shared folder in CASPER for each agency to view their demographic and quality measure data prior to public posting on the Home Health Compare website.

Accessing Preview Reports

1. Log into CASPER via the OASIS Welcome Page.
2. Select Folder Tab.
3. Select the Shared Folder Link which displays as: *State ID HHA Agency ID. For example, *IA HHA HLISA01.
4. Select Report link for viewing.

CMS modified the timeframe for the data reported on Home Health Compare to align with the new DRA reporting timeframe. The Home Health Compare data is refreshed at the end of each quarter.

For more information and for specific refresh dates for 2007, access website: http://www.cms.hhs.gov/HomeHealthQualityInits/08_HHQIReportingforAPU.asp#TopOfPage

» CMS Home Health Pay for Performance Demonstration

Purpose: To determine the impact of offering incentive payments to agencies for improving the quality of care rendered to Medicare beneficiaries, when such quality of care results in reduced need for additional services and consequently, reduced cost. It is budget neutral, meaning that incentive funds will be generated from within current spending levels ("Home Health P4P", 2006).

Eight proposed home health performance measures and weights

Incidence of:

1. Acute care hospitalization (25 points)
2. Incidence of emergent care (15 points)

Improvement in:

3. Bathing	(10 points)
4. Ambulation	(10 points)
5. Transferring	(10 points)
6. Urinary incontinence	(10 points)
7. Management of oral medications	(10 points)
8. Status of surgical wounds	(10 points)

Final design: Completed in early 2007 (other measures may be added)
Solicitation and recruitment for participation: Spring & summer 2007; participation is voluntary.
Demonstration timeline: October 2007 to September 2009
Scoring rules: For each measure, agencies in the top 20% in performance level and those in the top 20% with the greatest improvement qualify for the incentive payment. One agency cannot receive payment for both. Incentives for reaching performance levels will be larger than the reward for improvement.

For more information, access website: http://www.cms.hhs.gov/DemoProjectsEvalRpts/downloads/HHPP_Presentation.pdf

» Home Health Quality Improvement National Campaign

Centers for Medicare and Medicaid Services (CMS) and the Home Health Quality Improvement Organization Support Center (HHQIOSC) launched this campaign in January 2007 ("HHQI National", 2007).
National Goal: Patients receiving home health care will remain in their home setting and require fewer avoidable hospitalizations. Agency participation is voluntary.
Goal of Participating Agencies: To reduce the average acute care hospitalization (ACH) rate across all participating agencies by a 5% relative improvement from baseline to the end of the campaign. Each agency's improvement is measured relative to its own baseline.
Timeline:
March 2007: Posting of ACH risk-adjusted agency level baseline rates to Home Health Compare website. Baseline rates are taken from the 12-month period ending September 30, 2006.
February 2008: Re-measurement of rates from the 12-month period ending on February 28, 2008.
May 2008: Re-measurement rates made available to campaign participants.

For more information, access website: http://www.homehealthquality.org/hh/hha/default.aspx

» Home Health Quality Measures

Also known as: Home Health Compare
Origin: These measures are collected via the OASIS data set (USDHHS, "Home Health").
Goal: To improve care quality outcomes of Medicare certified home health agencies.
Endorsed by: National Quality Forum

These measures below are written as:
What the public sees on the CMS Home Health Compare website, followed by: *(What the agency sees on OBQI Risk-Adjusted Outcome Report)*

Percentage of patients who:

1. Get better in walking or moving around
   (Improvement in ambulation)
2. Get better at getting in and out of bed
   (Improvement in transferring)
3. Who have less pain when moving around
   (Improvement in pain interfering with activity)
4. Whose bladder control improves
   (Improvement in urinary incontinence)
5. Get better at bathing
   (Improvement in bathing)
6. Get better at taking their medicines correctly (by mouth)
   (Improvement in the management of oral medications)
7. Are short of breath less often
   (Improvement in dyspnea)
8. Stay at home after a homecare episode ends
   (Discharge to community)
9. Had to be admitted to the hospital
   (Acute care hospitalization)
10. Need urgent, unplanned medical care
   (Emergent care)

» Quality Measures of other Healthcare Providers

Being knowledgeable of other providers' quality measures gives home health the basis upon which to form alliances across healthcare settings to jointly improve specific outcomes, control cost, and increase market share. These include:

- Physician Quality Measures
- Hospital Quality Measures
- Nursing Home Quality Measures

» Physician Quality Measures/ Physician Quality Reporting Initiative

CMS 2007 Physician Quality Reporting Initiative (PQRI) has replaced the 2006 Physician Voluntary Reporting Program (PVRP) as a first step toward pay-for-performance for physician services. The latest physician quality measures statements were effective January 1, 2007. Eligible professionals who successfully report designated quality measures on claims from July 1 to December 31, 2007 may earn a bonus payment, subject to a cap, of 1.5% of total allowed charges for covered Medicare physician fee schedule services.

The proposed 2008 quality measures set must be published by August 15, 2007, and finalized by November 15, 2007.
Origin: Physician records
Goal: Substantially improve the health and function of CMS beneficiaries by preventing chronic disease complications, avoiding preventable hospitalizations, and improving the quality of care delivered.
Endorsed by: National Quality Forum (NQF), Ambulatory Care Quality Alliance (ACQA) and the American Medical Association (AMA).

The list below includes those measures that have strong application to home health patient assessment and care:

- For Type 1 or 2 Diabetes Mellitus
  - Hemoglobin A1c control
  - Low density lipoprotein control
  - High blood pressure control
- For CHF (left ventricular systolic dysfunction)
  - ACE Inhibitor or Angiotensin Receptor Blocker therapy
  - Beta blocker therapy
- For those with prior heart attack
  - Beta blocker therapy
- Antiplatelet therapy for those with coronary artery disease
- For stroke and stroke rehabilitation
  - Patient discharged on antiplatelet therapy
  - Anticoagulant therapy prescribed for atrial fibrillation at d/c
  - Screening for dysphagia
  - Consideration of rehabilitation services
- For osteoporosis
  - Communication with physician managing ongoing care post fracture
  - Management following fracture
  - Pharmacologic therapy
  - Counseling for Vitamin D, calcium intake and exercise
- Screening for fall risk
- Medication reconciliation

- Urinary Incontinence in women 65 years and older
  - Assessment of presence or absence of
  - Characterization of
  - Plan of care for
- Electrocardiogram for syncope
- For community-acquired pneumonia
  - Assessment of oxygen saturation
  - Assessment of vital signs
  - Assessment of mental status

For the latest updates on PQRI, access website:
http://www.cms.hhs.gov/PQRI
For the complete listing of all physician quality measures, access website: http://www.cms.hhs.gov/PQRI/Downloads/PVRPQualityMeasuresList.pdf

---

» Hospital Quality Measures

Also known as: Hospital Compare
Origin: Medical information from patient records are converted into a rate or percentage that shows how well hospitals provide care for some, but not all of their patients. (USDHHS, "Hospital Compare").
Goal: To distribute hospital performance data that encourages consumers and physicians to select the best hospital care, to create incentives for hospitals to improve care, and to support public accountability.
Endorsed by: Hospital Quality Alliance (HQA), American Hospital Association (AHA), Federation of American Hospitals, Association of American Medical Colleges and the Agency for Healthcare Research and Quality (AHRQ).

Access latest hospital quality measures at website:
www.hospitalcompare.hhs.gov/Hospital/Static/AboutHospQuality.asp?dest=NAV|Home|About|?QualityMeasures#TabTop

The Hospital Quality Measures include:
1. Eight measures for heart attack care
2. Four measures for heart failure care
3. Six measures for pneumonia care
4. Two measures for preventing surgical infections

Measures for Heart Attack Care
Percentage of patients who receive:
1. Aspirin at discharge
2. Beta-blocker at arrival
3. Beta-blocker at discharge
4. ACE Inhibitor or Angiotensin Receptor Blocker for left ventricular systolic dysfunction
5. Smoking cessation advice/ counseling
6. Thrombolytic agent received within 30 min of arrival
7. Percutaneous Coronary Intervention within 120 min of arrival

Measures for Heart Failure Care
Percentage of patients who receive:
1. Left ventricular function assessment
2. ACE inhibitor or Angiotensin Receptor Blocker for left ventricular systolic dysfunction.
3. Comprehensive discharge instructions
4. Smoking cessation advice/counseling

Measures for Pneumonia Care
Percentage of patients who receive:
1. Oxygenation assessment
2. Pneumococcal vaccination assessment and if applicable, vaccine
3. Blood culture before first antibiotic
4. Most appropriate initial antibiotic
5. Initial antibiotic within 4 hours of arrival
6. Smoking cessation advice/counseling

Measures for Preventing Surgical Infection
Percentage of surgery patients who receive:
1. Prophylactic antibiotic within 1 hour prior to surgical incision
2. Discontinuation of antibiotics within 24 hours after surgery end time

» Nursing Home Quality Measures

Also known as: Nursing Home Compare
Origin: The nursing home quality measures come from resident assessment data, the Minimum Data Set that nursing homes routinely collect on the residents at specified intervals during their stay.
Goal: To provide consumer and provider information on the quality of care in nursing homes that are Medicare and Medicaid certified and to help nursing homes with quality of care improvements.
Endorsed by: National Quality Forum (NQF) and nursing home industry stakeholders.

Access latest nursing home quality measures at website: www.cms.hhs.gov/NursingHomeQualityInits/10_NHQIQualityMeasures.asp#TopOfPage

Nursing Home Quality Measures include those for:
1. Long-Stay Residents
2. Short-Stay Residents

Measures for Long-Stay Residents
Percentage of long term residents who:
1. Receive flu vaccine during flu season
2. Are assessed and receive pnuemococcal vaccine
3. Have an increased need for help with daily activities
4. Have moderate to severe pain
5. Are high risk for and have pressure sores
6. Are low risk for and have pressure sores
7. Were physically restrained
8. Are more depressed or anxious
9. Lose control of bowels or bladder
10. Have/had catheter inserted and left in the bladder
11. Spent most of the time in bed or chair
12. Became worse in their ability to move about in and around their room
13. Lose too much weight
14. Have/had a urinary tract infection

Measures for Short-Stay Residents
Percentage of short-stay residents:
1. Who were given flu vaccine during flu season
2. Who were assessed for and given pneumococcal vaccine if needed
3. With delirium
4. Who had moderate to severe pain
5. With pressure sores

» Medicaid and SCHIP Quality Practices
(SCHIP: State Children's Health Insurance Program)

CMS is responsible for supporting State Medicaid and SCHIP programs in their efforts to achieve safe, effective, efficient, patient-centered, timely and equitable care. CMS will partner with States to share best practices, provide technical assistance to improve performance measurement, evaluate current improvement efforts to inform future activities, collaborate with quality partners and coordinate Center activities to ensure efficiency of operations (USDHHS, "Overview. Medicaid"). Considering how home health can be a part of this initiative can lead to an offering of new services.

For more information, access website:
http://www.cms.hhs.gov/MedicaidSCHIPQualPrac/01_Overview.asp

CMS Medicaid/SCHIP Quality Strategy includes the following:
- Evidence-based Care and Quality Measurement
- Payment Aligned with Quality
- Health Information Technology
- Partnerships
- Information Dissemination, Technical Assistance, and sharing of best practices.

• Evidence-Based Care and Quality Measurement
CMS supports states in their efforts to improve performance measurement and ultimately the quality of care through the use of evidence-based measure sets that have wide acceptability in the healthcare industry.

• Payment Aligned with Quality
Quality-based purchasing, also known as pay-for-performance, is a quality improvement and reimbursement methodology which is aimed at moving towards payments that create much stronger financial support for patient focused, high value care. Pay-for-performance attempts to promote reimbursement for quality, access efficiency, and successful outcomes. CMS supports states in their efforts to implement P4P programs.

• Health Information Technology (HIT)
HHS currently has a 10-year plan to transform the delivery of health care by building a new health information infrastructure, including electronic health records and a new network to link health records nationwide. CMS encourages states to explore creative uses of health information technology in their Medicaid and SCHIP Programs.

• Information Dissemination and Technical Assistance
CMS facilitates the sharing of model practices, lessons learned and innovative approaches to emerging issues through issues briefs, analysis of demonstration evaluations, participating in conferences, Web casts and other methods.

Notes

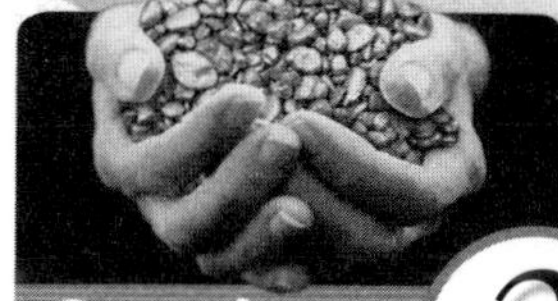

Section 2

Solutions for Success

» Staying Abreast of Changes in Healthcare

Staying abreast of trends that affect the home health industry gives agency executives better insight to determine future business strategy, sales and marketing plans, care provision, outcomes management, and technology needs. Most prominent are (in no particular order):

- CMS Quality Initiatives/P4P across all healthcare settings
- Medicare's initiatives for Value-Based Purchasing of Healthcare
- CMS focus on prevention and wellness- focus on vaccinations, seniors with multiple chronic conditions
- Obesity- has doubled in the Medicare population since '87, medical spending to treat Medicare beneficiaries has almost tripled.
- Shift to consumer-driven healthcare- Consumers are being given provider outcomes, health information and more responsibility for their own healthcare decisions.
- Continued rise in number of uninsured
- Well-educated, discriminating and demanding baby boomers
- Hospital-At-Home Care
- Electronic Health record and Web-based technology
- Remote patient monitoring
- Immigration
- Culture of Quality

» Institute of Medicine (IOM) Six Aims for Improving Healthcare in the U.S.

As your agency strives to improve quality outcomes while decreasing costs, be cognizant of how your projects fall in line with the Institute of Medicine's aims for improving healthcare in the U.S. The IOM (Institute of Medicine, "About") describes these as:

1. **Safe:** Avoid patient injury from care intended to help.
2. **Effective:** Provide evidence-based services to all who can benefit; refrain from those not likely to benefit.
3. **Patient-centered:** Respect and respond to patient preferences, needs, values, and have patient values guide all clinical decisions.
4. **Timely:** Reduce waiting and harmful delays for those receiving and giving care.
5. **Efficient:** Avoid waste of equipment, supplies, ideas and energy.
6. **Equitable:** Provide same care quality to all.

» Reducing Acute Care Hospitalization (ACH)

Intentional strategies used by the top ten percent of agencies who were most successful at reducing ACH and percent of agencies using the strategy (Briggs, 2006). Acute care hospitalization rates are posted on CMS Home Health Compare website quarterly.

1. 66% Fall Prevention
2. 64% Front Loading of visits
3. 61% Management culture and support
4. 59% 24 hr Availability/Response
5. 59% Medication Management
6. 52% Case Management
7. 48% Patient/caregiver education
8. 47% Special support services
9. 38% Disease management
10. 37% Physician relationships
11. 36% Data driven strategies
12. 33% Safety and risk assessment
13. 20% Hospital relationships with discharge planning staff
14. 8% Hospital relationships with emergency room staff
15. 8% Telehealth

To read the Briggs National Quality Improvement/Hospitalization Reduction Study in its entirety, access the website: http://www.nahc.org/NAHC/CaringComm/eNAHCReport/datacharts/hospredstudy.pdf

» OASIS Outcomes and Clinician Assessment Accuracy

Three factors affect OASIS outcomes:
1. Clinician accuracy in obtaining and documenting patient responses
2. Care delivery
3. Natural progression of patient's condition

It's imperative that home health clinicians who complete the OASIS instrument be knowledgeable of the definitions for all OASIS assessment items. Agencies must insure that clinicians know how to accurately obtain patient responses to the OASIS instrument, according to OASIS guidance found in the CMS OASIS User's Manual. Definitions and instructions for accurate assessment are located in Chapter 8 of the manual. The manual is available for download.

Access website: www.cms.hhs.gov/HomeHealthQualityInits/14_HHQIOASISUserManual.asp#TopOfPage

» OASIS Accuracy and Reducing Acute Care Hospitalization

There are two OASIS items that affect the agency's acute care hospitalization rate.
1. OASIS Item M0100: Reason for Assessment, Item #6 and Item #7
2. OASIS Item M0855: To which Inpatient Facility has the patient been admitted? Item #1

Guidance from the OASIS User's Manual:

<u>M0100: Reason for the Assessment</u>

1. Item#6: Transferred to an inpatient facility-patient not discharged from agency
   - Response used when patient is transferred to an inpatient facility for 24 hrs or longer (for reasons other than diagnostic tests).
   - Patient expected to resume care and is NOT discharged from the agency.
   - A home visit is not required. Data may gathered over the phone.

2. Item#7: Transferred to an inpatient facility-patient discharged from agency
   - Response used when patient is transferred to an inpatient facility for 24 hrs or longer (for reasons other than diagnostic tests).
   - Patient is discharged from the agency.
   - A home visit is not required. Data may be gathered over the phone.

» Clinician Accuracy and Reducing Acute Care Hospitalization

OASIS assessment strategies:

- If unsure as to the specific type of facility the patient is transferred to, contact the facility and ask what type of bed the patient has been admitted to, i.e., hospital bed, swing bed, or nursing home bed.
- If the patient is never admitted, but held in ER and stays longer than 24 hrs, this is classified as emergent care. Verify that patient was not admitted.

M0855: To which inpatient facility has the patient been admitted?
Because facilities may have different bed types, it's critical to select the correct bed to which the patient is admitted. You may contact the facility to inquire.

- Item 1 Hospital: an acute care bed
- Item 2 Rehabilitation facility: freestanding rehabilitation hospital, Rehab Unit of acute care hospital
- Item 3 Nursing Home: Skilled nursing facility (SNF), Intermediate care facility for mentally retarded (ICF/MR), or nursing facility (NF).
- Item 4 Hospice
- NA No inpatient facility admission

Access the OASIS User Manual at website: http://www.cms.hhs.gov/HomeHealthQualityInits/14_HHQIOASISUserManual.asp#TopOfPage

» Making the Most of Home Health Compare

One very effective method of using Home Health Compare outcomes is to:

1. Go to website.
2. Select all the agencies in your service area.
3. Study and compare findings.
4. Compare your agency to major competitors.
5. Make graphs that highlight the positives.
6. Use graphs to explain how you are addressing the negatives.
7. Be able to explain why percentages are what they are.
8. Be able to specify what the agency is doing that has affected percentages.
9. Note the outcome percentage differences over time.
10. Make graphs that reflect percentages over time.
11. Use graphs as appropriate to market your services to the public and referral sources or to enhance a referral source relationship.
12. Plan to periodically provide graphs with discussion.

Access Home Health Compare at website: http://www.medicare.gov/HHCompare/Home.asp

» Home Health Episode Management

Episode management generally describes a method used by home health providers to periodically review a 60-day episode of care. It may include OASIS accuracy, proper ICD-9 coding, projected therapy utilization and follow-up, supply use, projected reimbursement, and the HHRG relative to visits and the plan of care. The following questions are especially helpful in guiding home health episode management.
Note: For a complimentary Episode Management Tool, email your request to: info@outcome-architects.com

OASIS Accuracy

- Was the assessment submitted within regulatory/agency approved timeframe?
- Is the assessment complete?
- Are there incongruent OASIS responses?
- Do we know the agency's % of OASIS data entry error?

ICD-9 Coding

- Are the codes appropriate to the chief reason for the episode of care?
- Are codes supported by medical record documentation?
- Is the correct coding sequence used?
- Is coding to the highest degree of specificity?
- Is there correct use of additional codes, manifestation codes, and "code first" notes?
- Are correct codes used for case mix diagnoses?
- Are V-codes used correctly?

Care Coordination

- Is there a clearly defined process?
- Is the process working?
- How does the process support agency episode management?
- Are disciplines coordinating care with each other?

Resource Utilization

- Disciplines
  - Is discipline use appropriate?
  - Is there unnecessary use of disciplines?
  - Is discipline use in line with OASIS responses?
  - What is the process for follow-up of therapy visits?
    - Tips to monitor therapy use
    - - Conduct baseline audit: % of patients with/without therapy.
    - - Determine average visits made.
    - - Drill down reasons for adjustments.
    - - Determine dollars lost/appropriate to care.
    - - Audit the clinical record for plan of care implementation.
- Visits
  - Is the number of visits ordered congruent with patient need?
  - Is the number of visits appropriate to the HHRG?
  - Do discipline visits overlap unnecessarily?
  - Are patients satisfied with visits planned?
- Supplies
  - Are the type and number of supplies used appropriate to patient need? To use of evidence-based practice? For example, is moist wound treatment ordered for pressure ulcers?

» The Joint Commission 2007 Home Care National Patient Safety Goals

Note: The Joint Commission on Accreditation of Healthcare Organizations has changed their brand name from "JCAHO", commonly pronounced "Jayco" by healthcare providers, to "The Joint Commission".

The Joint Commission Home Care National Patient Safety Goals are requirements that pertain to the delivery of patient care in hospitals, homecare, ambulatory care and office-based surgery, assisted living centers, behavioral health, laboratory, long term care and networks ("The Joint Commission", 2007).

Goal: To promote specific improvements in patient safety.
Endorsed by: The Joint Commission and the Sentinel Event Advisory Group, who conducts an annual, systematic review of the literature to identify new goals and requirements.

Access more information about The Joint Commission's National Patient Safety Goals at website:
www.jointcommission.org/PatientSafety/NationalPatientSafetyGoals/
Note: Not all National Patient Safety Goals are pertinent to every healthcare setting. Only certain patient safety goals pertain to home health from the full set. The number below corresponds with the Goal Number in the full set, thus you will notice numbers out of sequence.

Home Care National Patient Safety Goals are:

1. Improve accuracy of patient identification
2. Improve effectiveness of communication among caregivers
3. Improve the safety of using medications
7. Reduce risk of healthcare-associated infections
8. Accurately and completely reconcile medications across the continuum of care
9. Reduce the risk of patient harm resulting from falls
13. Encourage patients' active involvement in their own care as a patient safety strategy
15. Organization identifies safety risks inherent in its patient population

» Using Evidence-based Practice to Improve Outcomes

A CMS premise for pay-for-performance is to reduce clinical practice variation. This speaks to standardization; whereby medical/nursing evidence is used consistently by physicians and clinicians with the purpose of improving outcomes of populations with chronic conditions. Standardization does not imply that every intervention is provided for every patient every time. Some interventions may not be applicable for the patient.

Evidence-based practice interventions that are based on healthcare research includes those provided by national associations and organizations, such as the American Heart Association, American College of Cardiology, American Diabetes Association, National Council on Aging, and the Wound, Ostomy and Continence Nurse Society, to name a few. For example, the new recommendation for hypertension is to obtain an accurate blood pressure reading; one that can be enhanced by having the patient avoid exercise, caffeine and smoking for 30 minutes prior to taking the reading (National Institutes of Health, "Seventh Report"). The application of this evidence-based practice intervention can help improve accuracy of the reading, which can in turn allow the physician to more aptly treat the diagnosis.

Note: See Section 5 of *Gold Nuggets* for a listing of websites that has evidence-based practice interventions and guidelines for use. For evidence-based DM outcomes and intervention tools for chronic conditions, e-mail: info@outcome-architects.com

» Using Cause and Effect to Improve Outcomes

Realizing that OBQI outcomes result in part due to the natural progression of disease, one should focus on the factors or causes that the agency can change that also affect these patient outcomes. The Cause and Effect diagram is a simple performance improvement tool that can be extremely helpful in identifying and exploring possible causes of a specific problem or outcome. Using a Cause and Effect Diagram is also a successful method for documenting your efforts and demonstrating performance improvement analysis that is conducted for the accreditation process.

10 Key Steps in Developing a Cause and Effect Diagram

1. Identify the main problem or outcome that needs remedy or reinforcement.
2. Form a small group of people whose line of work place them "closest to the problem" to brainstorm all possible causes.
3. List each cause given by the group.
4. Place each cause into one of four following categories:
   - Man
   - Machine
   - Method
   - Material
5. For each cause, ask "Why does this happen?" List the responses that apply to each cause directly below it.
6. Interpret findings.
   - Look for causes that occur repeatedly.
   - Determine how often causes occur.
   - Prioritize these items accordingly.
   - Specify the cause(s) for which the greatest impact can be realized.
   - Reach agreement among group members.
   - Seek to cure the cause, not the symptoms.
7. Decide upon the process, procedure, policy, etc. to address the cause(s) identified.
8. Educate all directly involved. Inform all others.
9. Implement.
10. Re-evaluate outcome or problem. Improved? Worsened? Remained same? Ask Why. Decide next course of action.

» Patient Outcomes of Knowledge and Compliance

Measuring additional patient outcomes, i.e., supplemental outcomes of knowledge and compliance, helps give perspective to the OASIS outcomes achieved.

Example: Ascertaining what the patient knows to do to prevent an exacerbation and what the patient does to prevent it can be important keys to achieving improvement in the OASIS outcome of ACH rate. Aside from the natural progression of the patient's condition, it's critical to measure a patient's knowledge of how to recognize and manage symptoms that signal him/her to action. Measuring this outcome gives perspective to the acute care hospitalization rate achieved. If the outcome of a population of patients shows that the rate of ACH is high, and the knowledge outcome is low, the agency then has a place from which to begin a meaningful investigation. Lack of knowledge could be a contributing factor to the ACH rate. If a knowledge outcome is not measured, then we don't know if there is a lack of knowledge or not that can affect the ACH rate.

To incorporate the use of knowledge and compliance outcomes, the agency must have a consistent process by which to measure and aggregate the outcome results. An agency can develop their own or purchase outcome-based documentation systems that include these outcomes. Either method should have outcomes written in such a way that the user understands what is being measured, how to measure it, and when to measure it.

Examples: Goals that the nurse measures as outcomes met, not met, or not applicable:

1. Patient/caregiver knows how to independently test own blood glucose by discharge. (The agency has a specific procedure that outlines the "have-to-know" steps the patient must take in order to test own blood glucose independently.)

2. Patient/caregiver is independent with managing wound by visit 9. (The agency has an outline of wound management that the nurse must address with the patient and caregiver(s). It includes priority items of assessing the wound for infection, cleansing the wound, dressing the wound, and waste disposal)

Another method of outcome measurement is provided by the University of Iowa, in a published document entitled, Iowa Outcomes Project: Nursing Outcomes Classification (Johnson, Maas, and Moorehead, 2000). Outcomes are measured on a continuum rather than as discrete met or not met goals.

Example: Extent of understanding conveyed about Diabetes Mellitus and its control

1. Indicator # 182014: Demonstration of the correct procedure for blood glucose testing

None	Limited	Moderate	Substantial	Extensive
1	2	3	4	5

» Developing a Home Health Specialty Rehabilitation Program

Several of the Home Health Compare Outcomes are a direct measurement of a patient's independence to perform certain tasks. These include: bathing, ambulation, transferring, and managing oral medications. Several studies indicate that providing specific, standardized protocols can enhance patient function and lead to improved outcomes. Therapists can also have a great impact on fall prevention through gait and balance training, and strengthening.

Steps to Establish a Rehab Specialty Program

1. Select a person to coordinate all aspects of the project on a daily basis and to keep momentum sustained. This person should have a general understanding of therapy interventions and outcomes management. He/she should have a keen knowledge of office policy and procedure.
2. Have key leadership staff, as well as those who will market the program, involved in the initial discussion about offering this new service. Include quality management, staff development, and the Director(s). Include senior rehab staff as appropriate for your organization.
3. Discuss how this program can affect the agency's quality outcomes business plan and marketing strategy.
4. Include fall prevention as a clinical strategy and as a community outreach program for older adults.
5. Consider agency outcomes in addition to Home Health Compare outcomes that you may want to measure. For example, compliance with home exercise program, measurements from Tinetti balance, and fall and injury/outcomes. Keep the number of additional outcomes small and manageable.

6. Choose the instruments to collect data. For example, a specific outcomes collection tool, a pathway, a protocol, or choose a process whereby data is collected from the therapy evaluation and/or visit note.
7. Develop the data collection process. Quality management should oversee this process on a regular basis.
8. Select the individuals who will routinely analyze outcomes. Select therapists to be involved in the analysis on a periodic basis.
9. Educate and train staff.
10. Set a timeline for use of tool(s) on a trial basis and have therapists use for at least one-two weeks.
11. Discuss and decide upon a marketing plan.
12. Implement trial use of the program.
13. Revise policy, procedure, outcomes tools, and/or process accordingly.
14. Re-educate staff as needed.
15. Implement program and marketing plan.
16. Analyze outcomes monthly for three months to determine if measurements are correctly made and entered into the measurement system, if interventions are provided as agency intends, and if staff understands their role in helping to achieve outcomes.
17. Decide on monthly or quarterly outcomes aggregation and trending for agency outcomes (those in addition to Home Health Compare). Large organizations may find monthly aggregation easier to manage, while smaller agencies may find quarterly aggregation more effective.

» Transforming to an Outcome-based Agency Culture

The phrase "It always starts at the top" is especially true of changing an organization's culture or work environment. Pay-for-performance brings an added dimension to the need for transforming our work and work place. To successfully transform, we must first change our mindset from being a part of an organization that provides good patient care to one that provides good quality care, measures and shares the results of that quality, reduces costs, maintains patient satisfaction, increases market share, and retains competent staff.

Change efforts that can have a direct, positive impact on the bottom line have 6 key qualities in common ("Keys to successful change").

1. Strong buy-in at the top
2. Employees are centered on common values
3. Change initiatives are team-driven
4. Skills-based training is provided
5. Results are measured
6. Management sticks to the plan

Senior Management:

1. Believes in the task at hand and has input in or has developed the framework of the task.
2. Articulates the vision and desired end-result to all staff.
3. Supports the staff prior to and throughout the change by encouraging, explaining, clarifying, and disciplining if needed.
4. Conducts brief sessions periodically with all levels of staff to keep them informed of individual and agency progress.
5. Sees that appropriate education and training are made available to meet the learning needs of staff, and that staff are supported in their participation.
6. Introduces or participates in the education and training.
7. Helps to establish or approves measures to quantify results.
8. Evaluates whether the team is working effectively day to day. Recommends or makes adjustments as needed.
9. Recognizes, removes or lessens obstacles to progress.
10. Recognizes that successful change initiatives take time.

» Fall Prevention

Briggs 2006 National Quality Improvement/Hospitalization Reduction Study found that fall prevention was the number one strategy used by top performing agencies to reduce their acute care hospitalization rates. The author's work has revealed 10 tips for successful fall prevention:

1. Investigate all falls while patient is under a home health plan of care.
2. Use evidence-based fall risk assessment items.
3. Link fall occurrence to emergent care use and acute care hospitalization outcomes.
4. Determine number of falls with/without injury.
5. Use an incident report that asks key questions of the patient.
   - What were you doing at the time of the fall?
   - What do you believe caused the fall?
6. Use evidence-based practice interventions.
7. Provide staff education to both skilled and unskilled disciplines.
8. Use standardized patient teaching materials dedicated to preventing falls in older adults.
9. Market your program to referral sources.
10. Provide education through community outreach.

Note: For information about Home Care Fall Prevention: An Evidence-Based Program, contact the Briggs Corporation at 800.224.2187

» Winning Managed Care Over to Your Side

Working successfully with managed care requires more than solid interpersonal telephone skills. Success can be best realized when these relationships are based on joint outcomes of interest. When a managed care organization (MCO) understands that the agency is concerned with quality outcomes and costs, you immediately establish common ground. Home health programs that can demonstrate aggregation and trending of outcomes specific for chronic diagnoses and conditions can be the platform of a successful relationship.

1. Determine percentage of patients served under each contract you have.
2. Select contracts of high patient volume.
3. Review typical requirements for admission and subsequent visit verification.
4. Ask if organization has disease management (DM) or chronic condition programs they can share.
5. Evaluate appropriateness of their DM program interventions for your agency's patients.
6. Determine if your agency can provide DM interventions as outlined by the managed care organization.
7. Evaluate staff competency required to implement program(s).
8. Determine competencies needed.
9. Plan/conduct education and training.
10. Discuss outcomes of interest to the managed care group.
11. Determine the method by which these outcomes can be shared and how often.
12. Discuss change in requirements of admission and visit approval process.
13. Identify point person for monitoring and follow-up.

» Financial Outcomes to Monitor by Diagnosis & by Referral Source

Monitoring these outcomes by diagnosis and referral source helps an agency pinpoint areas where remediation efforts can have the greatest impact on quality and finance. Monitor these as an average for a prospective payment system (PPS) 60-day episode of care.

1. Average reimbursement
2. Average case mix
3. Visits by discipline
4. Visit costs by discipline
5. Visit costs by episode
6. Supply costs by episode
7. Profit/Loss (Reimbursement minus total cost of care)

» Winning with Chronic Wound Care

Your agency can attain quality outcomes by providing evidence-based wound care interventions. These interventions include risk assessment, nutrition, pressure relief, wound assessment, proper staging, moist wound treatment, and changing course promptly when treatment is not effective.

Establish a baseline of current agency wound care practice.

1. Determine type of wound care generally ordered by each physician/surgeon who admits to the agency.
2. Review agency policy, process and decision-making responsibility for procuring pressure relief devices and establishing nutrition needs on admission to the agency.
3. Look at the agency's OBQI wound outcomes over the last quarter and the last 12 months. These are:
   - Increase in pressure ulcers
   - ACH due to wound infection, deterioration or new lesion. **Note: Infections from tube sites are included here. Except these out of your evaluation.*
   - Emergent care due to wound infection, deterioration or new lesion.
   - Discharge to community needing wound care
4. Review a sample of charts and determine average days to healing outcome for wet-to-dry wound treatment and average to days to healing for moist wound treatment. **Note: "Days to healing" can be defined as the number of days required to heal the wound and/or number of days until caregivers independent with wound care.*

5. Determine average direct cost of agency's wet-to-dry wound treatment versus moist wound treatment.
   ***Note:** Moist wound treatment includes dressings such as hydrocolloids, foam, hydrofiber™, silver, etc. designed to keep the wound bed moist and undisturbed for days at a time.
   Real direct costs include (Ovington, 2001):
   - Price of the dressing
   - Other supplies and services, such as gloves, tape, biohazard waste containers, and disposal
   - Labor cost to change the dressing (include mileage, visit costs)
6. Compare findings for each physician, wound clinic, other referral source.
7. Prepare bar graphs of findings.
8. Determine how findings of each physician's wound treatment are affecting agency quality outcomes and costs.
9. Establish a wound products formulary with minimal choices for staff providing wound care.
10. Use wound product vendors to provide staff and physician education, and wound care tools.
11. Visit each physician and demonstrate how his/her wound treatment (quality and cost) compares with others.
12. Discuss positives and negatives.
13. Be prepared to offer a solution that includes the use of evidence-based moist wound treatment.

» Forming Alliances with Wound Care Vendors

Wound care vendors are rich with resources for their customers. Ask about:

- Evidence-based protocols
- Product selection guides
- Scientific research for physicians
- Staff education assistance
- Patient teaching materials
- Wound measurement tools
- Staging guides
- Guidance with a wound prevalence study

Wound product vendors typically assist in the development of the agency's wound product formulary. Establishing a product formulary helps to keep costs down and narrows the selection for users, making it easier to identify the most appropriate product according to patient need.

» Wound Prevalence Study

These studies give the agency a baseline that describes its wound patient population at a specific point in time. Wound prevalence is also used to guide agency leaders in prioritizing its wound populations of greatest need. When coupled with OBQI outcomes, wound prevalence data becomes powerful information for decision-making, outcomes management, staff development, an outcome-based collaborative, and business and marketing strategy.

A wound prevalence study includes a chart review of all patients with primary and secondary diagnoses of wounds. To determine wound prevalence in the agency's patient population, include at least the following data in the chart review:

1. Patient ID #
2. M0175 (Discharged from an inpatient facility?)
3. Age
4. Race
5. Gender
6. M0360 (Primary Caregiver)
7. M0370 (How often is assistance received?)
8. Number of wounds
9. Wound type, i.e., surgical, pressure, neuropathic, arterial, venous stasis
10. Wound size(s)
11. Wound stage (s)
12. Dressing type in current use, i.e., film, foam, occlusive, alginate, chemical debridement
13. M0520 (Urinary Incontinence)
14. M0540 (Bowel Incontinence Frequency)
15. Albumin level, if known

Determine percentages using the following formula:
Numerator: Number of the part in question
Denominator: Total number of parts making the whole

For example, at the time of the study, there are 50 patients with wounds. Eight patients have incontinence; 38 patients have pressure ulcers.

8 divided by 50 =16% of the agency's total wound population has incontinence.

38 divided by 50 = 76% of the agency's wound patients have pressure ulcers.

» Health Coaching to Enhance Patient Self-Management of Chronic Conditions

Health coaching gives health care providers a framework by which they can determine the issues, beliefs, and concerns that may hinder or support a person's lifestyle change or responsibility for health that lies ahead for the individual. The reason for health behavior change comes from the patient, which increases the likelihood that ambivalence toward the change will be replaced with readiness for change (Miller and Rollnick, 1990).

Health coaching replaces the traditional "Do as I say, because I have the answers for you" model of care and allows the patient to discover why he/she has any existing ambivalence to change. Coaching provides motivation, encouragement, and health education in an atmosphere where full attention is given to the patient and where self-discovery can be achieved.

Health coaching enlists a number of techniques, some of which are listed below (Huffman, 2007).

1. Start with what the patient says his goal or problem is relative to his/her health condition.
   Example: What concerns you the most about your condition?
2. Use open-ended questions.
   Example: What is the most important thing that home care can do for you related to your health concerns?
3. Uncover any obstacles to patient's progress.
   Example: What do you think would help you most to walk 30 minutes a day, 5-6 days/week?
4. Affirm patient's strengths.
   Example: You had an excellent idea of having your son call you in the evening to remind you to take your pill.
5. Use reflective listening.
   Example: You said that you have shortness of breath when going to the mailbox. Tell me more about this.
6. Summarize the conversation that has taken place.
   Example: We've talked about your concerns re: your shortness of breath and when you have the most difficulty, as well as conserving your energy throughout the day. We also talked about the shortness of breath scale that you agreed to use to describe these occurrences to the nurse.

» Competency Assessment (Evidence-based)

A competency assessment can be used to support and educate staff, and to prioritize those skills that are important for the clinician to master, related to patient populations for which evidence-based care is being provided. Use the evidence to help prioritize skills needed to manage patient populations of particular interest to the agency. It can include those skills that the agency deems necessary to provide a new service, to engage in a new referral relationship, or to achieve Home Health Compare outcomes, or other quality outcomes measured through a pathway or other process. Consider integrating the competency assessment score(s) or evaluation(s) in the employee's annual performance appraisal.
Competency of visiting staff must be assessed by qualified individuals.

1. Focus on those services, chronic conditions, or outcomes that the agency has determined a priority.
2. Select best practices that support these services, outcomes or patient care.
3. Research evidence-based practice guidelines for skills required.
4. Select those interventions that your staff has difficulty or anticipates difficulty with. Ask them.
5. Choose 1-2 items that agency deems of highest priority.
6. Decide how to measure this skill during the competency assessment.
7. Decide how often that competency testing will be conducted.
8. Review competency items at least annually to determine continued appropriateness for use.

» Performance Appraisal (Outcome-Based)

"Accepting mediocre performance yields an environment of mediocrity." Melinda Huffman

Using a P4P payment philosophy, develop a performance appraisal that rewards increases for staff contributions to the agency's achievement of outcomes. The appraisal becomes more objective than subjective. This requires an agency to adopt a philosophy that promotes a culture of quality and to move away from the concept of "raise across the board" mentality. This is much easier to envision in theory than to embrace in reality. It starts with leadership, of course! Think of this as investing in staff performance for higher returns in a pay-for-performance environment.

We have found the use of the following method to be exceptionally successful.

1. Determine agency categories of performance.
   Example: Quality, Quantity, Job Knowledge, Customer Service, Attendance, Behavior, Punctuality, and Appearance.
2. Prioritize category importance by deciding the percentage of 100 to give each category.
   Example: Quality may be given 35%, whereas Attendance may be given 2%.
3. Develop any number of appraisal items by category based primarily on outcomes.
   Example: Manages own workload to keep OT at < 3%.
   Agency ACH rate is at or below the national average.
   Demonstrates ability to independently manage agency's infusion protocol.
4. Select the number of performance levels the appraisal will have. Five levels are recommended.
   Example: Level 5 Exceptional
   Level 4 Above Average
   Level 3 Satisfactory
   Level 2 Below Average
   Level 1 Unsatisfactory
5. To "weight" each category according to the % given to each, determine the weight factor to apply to each category.
   Example: Quality 35%
   - 35% divided by the number of items in Quality = weight factor
   - Employee points attained in the category (X) weight factor = category points
   - Add all weighted category points. This equals the performance appraisal points attained.
6. Determine the number of points for each level that corresponds with the reward attained.
7. List all employees who rate satisfactory. These persons receive the "average" raise increase approved by Administration.
9. Remaining employees receive either higher rewards for stellar performance or no reward for lesser performance.
10. Rank employees according to reward attained. Use Excel to accomplish this task. The agency now has the number of employees who are "average" versus those who are above and below average. Figure these percentages.

Note: For guidance on developing a performance appraisal based on P4P payment methods, contact the author via e-mail: info@outcome-architects.com

» Disease Management

Disease Management (DM) is an approach to delivering health care to persons with chronic conditions that aims to improve patient outcomes while containing healthcare costs. The Disease Management Association of America states that a full service DM program should consist of six components. Programs that have less than six are referred to as support service providers (Disease Management Association of America, n.d.).

These six are:

1. Identification of chronic populations
2. Use of evidence-based practice interventions that have been found to improve quality outcomes
3. Patient/enrollee and family self-management education
4. Collaboration with physicians, care providers, support service providers
5. Outcome measurement, evaluation, and management
6. Routine feedback and reporting loop

Certain conditions are ideal for home health DM. Some of these are:

- Congestive Heart Failure
- Hypertension
- Coronary Artery Disease
- Obesity
- Asthma
- Chronic wounds
- Diabetes
- Depression
- Chronic Obstructive Pulmonary Disease

» Disease Management Action Plan for Home Health

1. Determine agency readiness for an outcome-based culture and for DM as a business strategy.
   - Identify DM program coordinator
   - Select or develop the system of implementing consistent evidence-based practice among clinicians
2. Prioritize and select DM patient population(s) through a variety of factors:
   - Large volume
   - Chronic diagnoses
   - Critical/New referral sources
   - Co-morbidities
   - Business strategy
3. Determine evidence-based practice that will be used and how.
4. Determine if new product formularies, supplies, and/or equipment are needed for the new service or program.
5. Determine the disciplines appropriate for providing care.
6. Define staff competencies that are needed.
7. Determine "best fit" technology for your agency and cost effectiveness.
8. Plan education and training.
9. Develop or select evidence-based patient teaching materials that support interventions provided.

9\. Contact DME and supply vendors to establish product formularies and pricing.

10\. Select OBQI outcomes for integration into DM approach. For example, Improvement in dyspnea for patients with CHF.

11\. Consider additional outcomes of patient knowledge and compliance to measure.

12\. Decide how these outcomes will be measured, aggregated and trended.

13\. Identify the persons or groups to include in your outcomes reporting and feedback loop.

14\. Select best method of sharing outcomes data.

15\. Conduct annual agency DM program evaluation and include in business plan.

16\. Plan outcome-based marketing strategies. Evaluate effectiveness.

» Common Features of Disease Management Organizations

Home health providers must know how Disease Management Organizations (DMOs) provide care to participants/enrollees in order to collaborate or compete in the new healthcare market. Generally, DMOs:

1. Target specific consumer populations with chronic conditions, such as obesity, CHF, Asthma, CAD, and Diabetes.
2. Use phone contacts from healthcare professionals to guide and instruct.
3. Provide personalized goal-setting and tracking.
4. Offer 24-hr call access to nurses.
5. Provide educational materials by mail, video or internet.
6. Conduct electronic monitoring of key vital signs or measures.
7. Provide updates and reminders to physicians.
8. Use clinical information systems to drive standards of care and evidence-based practice interventions.
9. May share data with physician via secure internet.
10. Receive payment on a per-member per-month (PMPM) basis, commonly with risks/incentives for results (Andersen, 2006).

» Selecting Agency "Best Fit" Technology

Golden rule of buying and using technology:
Use the technology you have to its maximum capability before purchasing more.

1. List the technology you have. Include phone and fax.
2. List what your technology is currently used for.
3. Review business plan and strategy in light of technology use and need.
4. Identify primary patient populations served.
5. Evaluate current management of supplies. Discuss how technology could help you manage supply use and costs more effectively. Call upon vendors to discuss if needed.
6. Prioritize clinical and financial outcomes that the agency will collect and monitor.
7. Determine if potential revenues are being lost that technology could rectify.
8. Investigate technology needs that will enhance agency alliance relationships, outcomes sharing, care efficiency, and information flow.
9. Evaluate ease of use as perceived by both staff and patient/caregiver, as appropriate.
10. Develop a realistic change management protocol to assist agency staff in transition from manual to automated processes. This is a common reason why technology implementations often do not go as well as intended.
11. Determine your return on investment prior to purchase.
12. Consider risk management issues. Read contract carefully. Ask questions. Know whose responsibility it is to respond when equipment fails, when alerts are sent out, and in what timeframe the response is expected.

» Telephone Nursing and Teletriage

Use your agency telephone to its maximum potential to help decrease acute care hospitalization. The Home Telehealth Reference 2007 is available for download from the Medicare Quality Improvement Community's website: www.medqic.org. Coordinated through Quality Insights of Pennsylvania, this valuable resource contains teletriage guidelines, routing of calls, teletriage competencies, physician education and decision support tools.

There are also established companies which provide telephony services that make and answer calls to patients that include questions and answers specific to the management of chronic conditions and general triage. A telephony package is purchased most appropriate to agency need. Several studies support the use of telephone nursing and give us insight into its success, as well as issues that should be considered when implementing a program of this kind. Greenburg and Schultz (2002) share several findings worthy of note:

Patients with chronic conditions call most frequently:

1. for the coordination of care and visits.
2. to maintain continuity of care.
3. to seek clarification from a physician or clinic visit.
4. to ask questions.

Other patients of all ages use the service most often to:

1. avoid calling the doctor's office.
2. ask about a prescription.
3. seek reassurance.
4. get advice about symptoms.
5. ask whether to seek care or provide self-care.

To promote patient satisfaction with telephone triage, consider the following issues that patients said were most important to them:

1. Timeliness of returned call
2. Timeliness of answered call
3. Identification and title of caller
4. Pleasant greeting
5. Value patient's input
6. Convenience and time-saver
7. Accurate information
8. Want to avoid clinic or doctor's office visits
9. Speak directly with nurse when call is placed
10. Call answered quickly by "real" person

» Measuring Return on Investment

Return on Investment (ROI) measures the financial return of an investment or the effectiveness of a project, like telemonitoring (TM). To determine the overall value, you must assess the purchase cost and the value it yields over time, along with the savings realized due to the purchase (Contino, 2004). The ROI for technology is not always easy to project, because there are gains that are difficult to measure.

Consider the following savings (Contino, 2004):
- Decreased supply/printing costs
- Fewer visits
- Projected life of equipment and replacement costs
- Improved efficiency
- Improved communication
- Projected life of equipment and replacement costs

The following formula may be helpful and can also be used to measure ROI by patient population, i.e., by ICD-9 code if you are considering using TM for a specific patient group, such as CHF.

ROI = Reimbursement(Revenue) - Cost

1. Determine current reimbursement (revenue) and costs for 12 months before and after implementation of TM. Construct a table for these comparisons.

Reimbursement (Revenue)
- Average reimbursement/episode
- Number of episodes/year
- Annual reimbursement revenue

Costs
- Average nurse cost/visit
- Average visits/episode
- Average nurse visit costs/episode
- Average miles/visit/episode
- Mileage rate per mile
- Average mileage cost/episode
- Annual nurse visit costs
- Number of monitors
- Annual monitor costs
- Annual maintenance fees, if applicable
- Total annual monitor equipment costs

- Number of staff required for TM
- Annual salaries dedicated to TM
- Total annual TM staff costs
- Annual TM costs
- TM Marketing costs (Training, Brochures, etc.)

Formulas

ROI

Reimbursement – Costs = profit or (loss) per episode; annually

Reimbursement revenue

(# of episodes [actual; projected] per year) X (Average reimbursement per episode) = Annual reimbursement revenue per year

Costs

(Avg nurse visit cost (Including benefits) X average visits/episode) + (Average miles/episode X mileage rate per mile) X (Episodes/year) = Annual visit costs (less patient supply costs)

Compare visit costs per episode with and without TM
Compare annual visit costs with and without TM

TM Costs = [(Number of monitors) X (monthly lease cost) X (12 months)] + (Annual TM staff salaries) + (Annual TM marketing costs) + (Annual maintenance fees, if applicable) = Annual TM costs

Compare Annual TM Costs to Annual Visit Cost Savings when TM in use.

Annual ROI

Annual Reimbursement Revenue - Annual Costs = Annual profit (loss)

Annual Profit (loss)

Annual Reimbursement Revenue = % Contribution Margin to fixed costs

» Outcome-Based Marketing Strategies

In an outcome-based healthcare environment, marketing efforts can best be realized when outcomes are the focus of getting and maintaining business relationships. In these strategies, healthcare outcomes become the primary reason the relationship is sustained.

1. Determine the outcomes that are of value to your referral source. Discuss how a joint approach through home health can improve these outcomes.
2. Focus on outcomes data relative to agency's special care/ treatment/services.
3. Provide one intake access number.
4. Provide referral sources with a customized, simple referral fax form.
5. Develop joint educational programs.
6. Provide community outreach services and programs.
7. Ask to participate periodically in hospital committee work relative to homecare.
8. Use competitor's Home Health Compare Data in comparison charts.
9. Network with physicians around office hours, i.e., special receptions, programs, lunch n' learn opportunities.
10. Share plans to improve outcomes of like interest.
11. Collaborate with hospitals to assist in decreasing their length of stay for CHF and use of emergency care.
12. Implement disease management programs.
13. Provide care plan oversight education.

» Collaborating with Physicians to Affect Cost and Quality

1. Determine the physicians whose practice patterns you want to influence because of cost or quality outcomes that are less than desired.
2. Determine change that is needed.
3. Conduct a chart audit on a sample of patients by each physician whose patients' outcomes you desire to improve, compared to a like physician whose desired outcomes are achieved.
4. Review patient outcomes of quality and cost.
5. Determine the cost of care and outcome percentages of care by physician.
6. Compare percentages by physician.
7. Develop graph(s) of findings.
8. Share findings with each physician as appropriate.
9. Use wound vendors to provide evidence-based data, if applicable, in support of a change in wound care practice.
10. Ask physician for a difficult patient to manage to demonstrate staff expertise.
11. Follow-up with physicians(s) on a regular basis to keep them informed of progress toward outcomes.

» Developing New Alliances to Achieve Quality Outcomes

Outcomes can be improved through strategic collaboration of parties who have a common interest in a particular outcome or set of outcomes. For example, a home care agency may improve the outcomes of emergent care use by collaborating with a local hospital that also shares this same desire. Together they determine how to approach the issue and may implement a joint approach or program to improve this outcome. They measure outcomes and share these findings on a periodic basis. This approach is also helpful when initiating a new service.

Eight Key Steps

1. Begin a dialogue with a referral source or other customer to identify the outcomes of special interest to them.
2. Establish specific patient populations of mutual interest by identifying particular needs of patient groups, according to volume.
3. Identify evidence-based practice interventions (EBP) likely to improve identified outcomes.
4. Identify existing gaps in the continuity of care between or among providers.
5. Determine if staff education and enhanced competency are needed to prepare your staff to implement interventions. Decide if alliance is best suited/has resources to help train agency staff.
6. Jointly develop patient and physician satisfaction indicators that will be measured.
7. Devise a plan for sharing outcomes and maximizing use of technology for efficient exchange of information.
8. Consider writing as a joint improvement initiative. Use in the accreditation process.

» Forming Alliances with Distributors

(Contributed by Ty Bello, President, TeamAtWork, LLC)

Distributors are generally wholesalers who act as intermediaries, and who sell or deliver products and supplies on behalf of the manufacturer to the retailer. Look beyond the immediate cost of the product and consider the total benefits of working with a distributor. Distributors can provide resources that will promote savings, accessibility, and a broad product offering.

1. **Customer Service:** Know how to communicate with your Customer Service Representative (CSR); hours of operation, e-mail, phone and fax numbers. Get the direct phone number of your CSR and use it!
2. **Distributor Sales Representatives:** Know how frequently the Sales Representative will be in touch with you. Establish your expectations up front.
3. **Manufacturer and Technical Support:** Categorize your products as *Frequently Used* and *Technical*. These are the products that will require the most support. Understand the line of communication and response time to these Manufacturers and Technical Support Teams.
4. **Primary and Alternate Shipping:** Know the location from where your products will be shipped and what the alternative shipping locations are in case of back order.
5. **Take the Guess Work out of Contract Negotiations:** View your distributor as a partner. Would you only provide partial information to a partner? This does not imply to give them current costing, but provide them with detailed product descriptions, volumes, and projected growth. This affords the most concise and reliable contract and pricing.
6. **Distribution Delivery Methods:** Distributors are most skilled in shipping products. Use this to your advantage. The fewer times a provider touches the product, the better. Ask if your distributor has Patient Direct or Patient Specific Shipping. Patient Direct goes directly to the patient, while Patient Specific goes to your facility specifically labeled for the patient, (no re-packing).
7. **Consider the use of a Distributor's Technology as Savings, not an Expense:** Ask your distributor about all of the technology they offer, i.e., EDI*, On-line Ordering, and Order Tracking. Investing in technology resources may very well demonstrate an overall savings that will more then pay for the investment. Ask them to assist with developing your ROI.

***EDI: See Section 3 for definition of Electronic Data Interchange**

» Networking to Grow your Business

An outcome-based healthcare environment is best served by networking with referral sources and other customers. Networking means giving value and receiving value from the relationship. Achieving desired healthcare outcomes can be a win-win for all parties.

Jeffrey Gitomer (2006), best-selling writer and speaker on sales and marketing, lists the following ways to make value-based networking happen.

You MUST:

1. Make and implement a strategic marketing plan
2. Earn mutual trust
3. Give value first
4. Be proactive in contacting and forming the relationship
5. Give first and give without "keeping score"
6. Allow time for these alliances to mature
7. Be creative about what you do and how you do it

» Remarkable Marketing

In Seth Goddin's acclaimed New York Times Bestseller, *Purple Cow,* he describes *remarkable marketing* as the art of building things worth noticing right into your product or service (Goddin, 2003). He tells the story of being enchanted by seeing hundreds of storybook cows grazing in the pastures on beautiful farms while driving through the countryside in France. As they drove, they continued to see this same picture mile after mile. After a while, seeing these cows no longer claimed his attention. They became boring. Very boring.... And he thought; "Now a purple cow would really get my attention".

From the author: I remember an experience of mine a several years ago while "marketing" our home care agency to a local hospital. After I explained the services and programs of our agency, the discharge planner looked at me and said, "What makes your agency programs different"? I was completely caught off guard. We had not taken a good look at ourselves and asked that same question.

Go to your website or look at your agency brochure. Notice the services listed. Many of the services are the same for many home health agencies: Nursing, Therapy, Home Health Aide, Hospice, Social Services, Dietician Services, In-Companion Care, and HomeMaker Services to name a few. These are important, but what truly makes your agency different, a purple cow? One that gets noticed.... One whose services are chosen over another? How can you transform your business into a purple cow? Into something remarkable? Review and evaluate your competitors' websites. Ask yourself the following questions:

1. How similar are they to your agency's website?
2. How different are they?
3. What would make me want to choose my agency over my competitor?

Consider your agency's strengths from an outcomes standpoint. Note your quality outcomes, specialty programs, financial outcomes and community outreach efforts. Also consider the alliances you have developed with your local hospital(s), physician groups, vendors or civic organizations. Develop ways of showcasing these features to agency customers.
Capitalize on the following items in your marketing campaign to showcase the value you bring to the patient and/or referral source:
1. Acute care hospitalization rate for chronic conditions below national or state average
2. Emergent care rate below national average
3. Fall with injury rate for older persons
4. % of patients whose wounds heal without complication
5. % of patients who become more functional through a special rehabilitation program

Changing your marketing efforts from explaining services to showcasing agency results allows your agency to differentiate itself from others. To be noticed as an agency that is special...as one that has something unique to offer...To be a purple cow...

» Helping Referral Sources Become and Stay Satisfied Beyond the Doughnuts!

While this list may seem obvious to some, it is not often that attention is paid to critical details in developing and maintaining a satisfied customer within a busy and hectic workweek. Take time during your next administrative/staff meeting to discuss these objectives, make your list, and set a timeline for executing your plan. This process is continual. We have found that incorporating these processes into the regular work of the organization enhances success:

1. Identify barriers to effective customer service as seen by the customer. Involve staff. Note complaints over the past year. Note phone calls from customers that have expressed concerns about service. Also consider performance improvement activities that originated from customer concerns about quality, timeliness, communication, and the like. Be critical during this self-evaluation.
2. List ways to overcome these barriers.
3. Suggest ways to create a positive relationship with customers. What do the customers want? Have we asked?
4. Discuss ways to improve communication with customers at all levels.
5. Formulate solutions. Always keep it simple when possible.
6. Communicate these efforts throughout the organization.
7. Evaluate success at a reasonable, specified time.
8. Revise as needed.
9. Continue this process.

» Healthcare Transformation and Home Health

Recognizing the challenges to success helps agencies keep a realistic perspective of the healthcare transformation underway and obstacles that must be eliminated or minimized. Andersen (2006) outlines several of these listed below that deserve thoughtful consideration. This transformation also affords home health new opportunities to achieve unparalleled success.

Challenges

1. Alignment of home health structure, processes and outcomes with healthcare system outcomes
2. Value of home health care is not well understood
3. New competitors entering the home health market
4. Lack of equal footing and integration with managed care
5. Investment in and adoption of innovative, proactive models of care
6. Developing new competencies
7. Adopting new technologies
8. Lack of sales and marketing skills
9. OASIS accuracy and coding
10. Financial resources

Opportunities

The transformation of healthcare affords the home health provider new opportunities to excel in achieving quality care outcomes and increased market share. Agencies are encouraged to seize opportunities and share their success. Some of these are listed below:

1. Strong focus of Medicare on home and community-based care
2. Use of outcomes data to elevate working relationships with managed care
3. Forming alliances with hospitals and disease management organizations
4. Studies have demonstrated cost effectiveness and quality of home health services
5. Providing participant education on behalf of Independent Practice Associations
6. Improving wound outcomes through vendor relationships and resources
7. Vendors and suppliers increasing their focus on home health
8. Basing partnerships on achieving outcomes of joint interest
9. Adapting evidence-based practice to the home health setting
10. Proactive requests for technology to ease home health documentation burden

11. Use of sales and marketing to grow business and to keep community/referral sources informed.
12. Increased need for community outreach to local populations with chronic conditions
13. Pay-for-performance transcending all healthcare settings
14. Use of outcomes generated through remote monitoring
15. Provision of hospice services and outcomes achieved for those at end-of-life
16. Grants for use of technology and for addressing the needs of underserved populations
17. New focus on prevention and screening for Medicaid populations

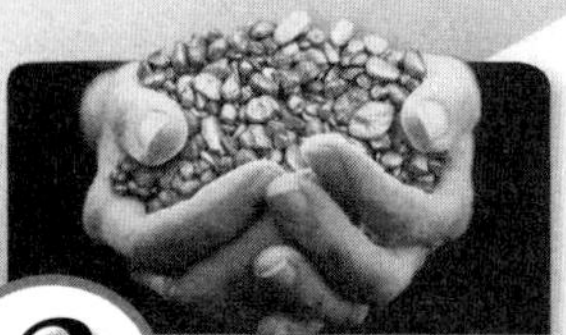

3 Section

Terms, Definitions & Examples

Subsection A
Home Health Disease Management, Outcomes, & Managed Care

» A

Adverse Event Outcome
An unusual or undesired patient occurrence that happens during the course of care (USDHHS, 2001). Outcome-based Quality Monitoring (QBQM) includes Adverse Event outcomes.

These are:
- Increase in pressure ulcers
- Development of UTI
- Unexpected nursing home admission
- Unexpected death
- Substantial decline in 3 or more ADLs (activities of daily living)
- Substantial decline in oral medication management

Adverse Event Outcomes Report
The Outcome Based Quality Monitoring (OBQM) Outcomes report that reflects potential problems in care because of their negative nature. (USDHHS, 2001). A home health agency is instructed to review all adverse event outcomes. The OBQM Adverse Event Outcomes Report is proprietary agency information.

Aggregate
A group or distinct mass gathered into a whole or considered as a total (Webster's New World College Dictionary, 1999).

Example: OASIS outcomes are aggregated into a whole at the national level to give agencies a benchmark by which to compare their own outcome results. Sometimes a total is referred to as an aggregate.

American Accreditation Commission (See URAC.)

Authorization
Permission given by the payer to a home health agency to allow visits and provide services.

Example: A managed care organization typically gives an authorization for home health visits throughout a patient's length of service prior to visits being approved for payment.

» B

Baseline (See also Benchmark, internal)
Internal data that serves as a starting point by which like data can be compared at a later point in time. This data can include clinical outcomes, financial outcomes, visit and supply utilization, patient demographics and the like.

Example: An agency wants to manage its visits more responsibly by decreasing the average visits per episode, while maintaining quality. Its current visit average is 22.6 visits per episode. This is the visit baseline that the agency will use to compare visits/episodes in the future.

Benchmark
The use of a point by which others are judged.
(Merriam-Webster, 2002).

Example: In home health, current external industry benchmarks are found in the Case Mix Profile Report, the OBQI Risk-adjusted and Descriptive Outcome Report and the OBQM Adverse Event Outcome Report.

Benchmark, Internal (See also Baseline)
Comparing one's own data at a specific point in time to same data collected at a later point or compared to same data of the company to which the agency is a part (Huffman, 2005b).

Example: An agency implements a quality improvement initiative through implementing evidence-based practice for Diabetes. The agency measures its patients' outcomes data as a benchmark before implementation and at a point in time afterward.

Benchmark, External
A point of reference or standard comparing one organization's performance with performance outside of the organization (JCAHO, 1994).

Example: Outcome-Based Quality Improvement (OBQI) provides a national reference within OBQI outcome reports that allows all home health agencies to benchmark their own outcome results against overall national outcomes.

Best Practices
Optimal techniques, procedures, or programs identified through evidence-based research or field experience of one or more organizations. Best practices are generally sought to improve care, thereby improving outcomes (USDHHS, 2006). Outcome-Based Quality Improvement (OBQI) in home health defines best practices as specific statements of clinical actions expected of staff in order to impact the problem, or strength identified in the statement.

Example: All patients with a primary diagnosis of hypertension will have blood pressure taken while seated and upon standing, every visit.

Briggs National Quality Improvement/ Hospital Reduction Study
A study sponsored by The Briggs Corporation in 2006 that focused on best practices used by the top ten percent of agencies who were most successful at reducing hospitalization rates, with a rate of 19% or lower (Briggs, 2006).

» C

Capitation
A method of payment for health services in which a practitioner or entity is pre-paid a fixed, per capita amount to cover a specific period of time for each person served, regardless of the actual number or nature of services provided to each person (Huntington, 1997).

Case Management
The process by which all health-related matters of a case, usually reserved for those cases that involve numerous providers and/or costly treatments, are managed by a health professional.

Case Mix
Patient's health status at home health admission and recertification that is based on responses for certain OASIS items (USDHHS, 2006).

Case Mix Profile Report
An OBQI report that shows demographics, characteristics, conditions, disabilities, and conditions of patients admitted to a home health agency within a specific time period, reported as percentages (USDHHS, 2006).

Care Plan Oversight
A billable service for physician supervision (not present) of a patient under the care of a home health agency or hospice that requires complex and multidisciplinary care modalities involving regular physician development and/or revision of care plans, review of subsequent reports of patient status, review of laboratory and other studies, communication (including phone calls) with other health care professionals involved in the patient's care, integration of new information into the medical treatment plan and/or adjustment of medical therapy, within a calendar month, of 30 minutes or more.

Access the following website for the complete listing of services that can and cannot be billed as care plan oversight: http://www.cms.hhs.gov/mcd/viewarticle.asp?article_id=33367&article_version=2&show=all

Chronic Condition
A disease that is characterized as one or more of the following: it is permanent, progressive if unmanaged, caused by non-reversible pathological alteration, requires special patient education for rehabilitation, self-monitoring, and self-management, and may require a long period of supervision, observation, or care (DMAA, 2004). Some chronic conditions include Heart Failure, Chronic Obstructive Pulmonary Disease, Diabetes Mellitus, Asthma, Obesity, Hypertension, Coronary Artery Disease, and End-Stage Renal Disease.

Clinical Practice Guideline
Systematically developed statements based on scientific methodology and expert clinical judgment that assist the practitioner to make patient decisions about health care for certain clinical conditions, with the purpose of improving clinical outcomes (USDHHS,1995).

Example: The Agency for Healthcare Research and Quality has developed a clinical practice guideline for the prevention and treatment of pressure ulcers in adults. It contains guidance in the areas of pressure ulcer risk assessment, skin care and early treatment, off loading and support surfaces, and education.

Compliance, Patient
The degree to which the patient follows health interventions as agreed with the health provider (Huffman, 2005a). Some literature suggests that compliance connotes a one-sided relationship. Therefore, more authors are beginning to use the terms, adherence and concordance. Adherence includes "being connected" or associated by contract, while concordance is described as an agreement between a patient and a healthcare professional about whether, when, and how prescriptions for health and well-being are taken.

Co-Morbidity
A secondary diagnosis or co-existing condition originating prior to admission for patient care and services that often complicates treatment for the primary condition, increasing costs and potential for complications (USDHHS, 2002).

Example: Hypertension is the most common co-morbidity seen in about 30% of all hospitalized patients. Other common co-morbidities are depression at 5% and obesity at 4%.

Community-Acquired Infection
An infection acquired from the general community or other members of the household. The infection is not associated with a discharge from an acute care setting or long term care facility and is not associated with the services rendered by a home care organization (McGoldrick, 2007).

Community Healthcare Accreditation Program (CHAP)
An independent, non-profit accrediting body that certifies that an organization has voluntarily met the highest standards of excellence for home and/or community-based health care.

Competency Assessment
The determination of an individual's capability to perform; with capability being assessed, demonstrated, and improved (JCAHO, 2006).

Competitive Bidding (Competitive acquisition)
Allows durable medical equipment (DME) suppliers to competitively bid for contracts with CMS to provide DME to a Medicare population.

Conditions of Participation
Federal regulations under which a home health agency is allowed to participate in Medicare and Medicaid programs (Ferris, 2006).

Consumer –Driven Health Care
In the context of group medical insurance:
Employee incentives to allocate his/her own medical dollars wisely.

Examples: The main types of plans under consideration in consumer-driven healthcare are (American Management Association, n.d.):

- Full-defined Contribution—The employee is responsible for finding and purchasing individual medical coverage. The employer provides funding through either direct compensation or a voucher.
- Tiered Networks—The employer offers employees a choice of medical plans, which include medical systems of varying costs.
- Menu-driven—Employers provide online information to help employees customize their own benefit plan by selecting co-pays, deductibles, etc.
- Managed Competition—The employer provides a subsidized basic medical plan with buy-up options. Plans can be from the same or multiple insurers.
- Health Savings Accounts—Current options include Medical Savings Accounts, Flexible Spending Accounts and Health Reimbursement Arrangements.
- Other options are still under Congressional consideration

Costs by discipline
Agency dollars spent per discipline in the provision of patient care (Huffman, 2005b).

Example: Cost by RN, cost by skilled nurse, cost by nursing, cost by physical therapy, cost by speech therapy and the like.

Culture, Agency/Organizational Quality
The personality of an organization consisting of values and operational standards that support members and their behaviors in striving for perfection (Quality Insights). CMS is encouraging home health agencies to develop a culture of quality to improve health outcomes.

» D

Data Quality
Data quality is synonymous with data integrity. It is the accuracy, consistency, and completeness of data. Data quality must be established prior to use.

Example: OBQI/OBQM outcomes data quality depends on OASIS assessment accuracy of the clinician.

Decision Support System
The organization of logically-related, computerized data that is used for decision-making to improve the quality and/or efficiency of patient care management (Sheyte and Struk, 2003). Decision support systems may be:
1. Purchased as part of a vendor's software package
2. Purchased as a separate framework
3. Developed by the agency

Demonstration Project
Studies financially supported in part or in whole by the federal government that are used to "test" various approaches to health care to improve quality and reduce costs.
Demonstration projects can be accessed via Medicare's website at:
www.cms.hhs.gov/DemoProjectsEvalRpts/

Direct Costs
The cost of care attributed to hands-on care and supplies used for the home visit, minus administrative overhead (Hagenow, 1999).

Example: The direct costs of wound care include the home health visit (labor) costs, supply costs, and mileage.

Disease Management (DM)
A system of coordinated health care interventions and communications for populations with conditions in which patient self-care efforts are significant (DMAA).

The DM approach consists of:
- Identification of specific populations
- Use of evidence-based practice guidelines
- Use of self-management education
- Collaboration among physicians, care providers, and support-service providers
- Outcome measurement, evaluation and management
- Routine reporting and feedback loop

Example: Disease management is offered by organizations and various providers, including home health, to control costs, focus on patient self-management and prevention, collaborate with physicians, and improve quality outcomes.

Disease Management/Outcomes Specialist
One who specializes in providing disease management resources, services, consultation and/or products to healthcare providers. CMS

recommends the use of DM specialists to support healthcare providers in the provision of chronic care (Huffman, 2006).
Access www.outcome-architects.com for more information about home health disease management consultation.

Disease Management Organization (DMO)
A DMO is an entity that provides disease management interventions for persons with chronic conditions. A DMO uses predictive modeling, pharmacy, medical and hospital claims, risk stratification, and return on investment as components of their approach to providing interventions (DMAA, 2004).

» E

Electronic Health Record (EHR) or **Electronic Medical Record** (EMR)
Patient health information that moves with the patient as he/she moves from one provider to another during the course of care or patient health information that is electronically stored and used by a single provider.

Example: Point of care (POC) devices store patient health information electronically for use by a home health provider. Some of these devices have electronic portals that allow the physician easy access to patient information needed for approval and signature.

End-Result Outcome (See OASIS outcome)

Enrollee, Managed Care
Person eligible for health plan services and benefits. Also referred to as member, subscriber, beneficiary (Huntington, 1997).

Episode of Care
PPS: A 60-day period of time for which home health reimbursement is generated. Reimbursement is based on the clinician's documentation of OASIS responses and is given for a single 60-day episode of care. Fifty percent is given after the Request for Anticipated Payment (RAP) is received and 50% at patient discharge, minus any adjustments throughout the episode (Medicare Payment Advisory Commission, 2005).

OBQI: The period of time from Start of Care to Discharge during which the completion of OASIS instruments generate outcomes for the patient.

Evidence-Based Practice
Using the best scientific evidence available to guide clinical decision making (DMAA, 2004).

Example: The use of evidence-based practice guidelines, evidence summaries and evidence reports to guide patient care interventions are considered the implementation of evidence-based practice.

Evidence Report
A report that delineates how evidence-based practice is used in the clinical area by providing an analysis of the scientific data, level of evidence and recommendations for clinical practice (Benefield, 2002).

Evidence Summary
An analysis of findings of multiple research studies that presents a state of the science conclusion (Benefield, 2002).

» F

Feedback Loop
Used in disease management to denote the groups or individuals who share outcomes data, communication, and other related outcomes information (Huffman, 2005b).

Example: An agency may collaborate with physicians, a local hospital, or clinic and include these providers, along with a patient group in their feedback loop.

FIM ™ Instrument
The FIM ™ Instrument is the most widely accepted functional assessment measure in use in the rehabilitation community. It is an 18-item ordinal scale, used with all diagnoses within a rehabilitation population. It is viewed as most useful for assessment of progress during a patient's rehabilitation.

For over 15 years, FIM was an acronym for "Functional Independence Measure". It is still often cited as such. However, Uniform Data System for Medical Rehabilitation, a division of UB Foundation Activities, Inc., states that the proper name is FIM™ Instrument, and should be referred to as such (van Hout communication, 2007). The FIM™ Instrument has become proprietary.

For further information on the FIM™, access website:
http://www.udsmr.org

Admission FIM™ Score is the baseline functional assessment done using the FIM™ Instrument at the time of admission to the rehabilitation program. The FIM™ Instrument should be administered within 72 hours after admission.
For the complete FIM System® Glossary, access website:
http://www.udsmr.org/fim2_gloss.php

Financial outcome
Data related to reimbursement and costs of patient care provision (Huffman, 2005c).

Examples: Home health financial outcomes include, but are not limited to:
- Average reimbursement by diagnosis
- Average visits per discipline
- Costs by discipline
- Discipline costs by diagnosis
- Average supply utilization
- Supply use by diagnosis
- Wound management costs

Financial Outcome Report
Financial data organized in a variety of ways that assists healthcare leadership to analyze and evaluate revenue and costs (Huffman, 2005c).

Example: Financial costs can be viewed in a spreadsheet format that includes all or some of the financial outcomes of interest to the agency.

Formulary
A collection of recipes, formulas and prescriptions (Dorland's, 2000). In home health, wound formularies are recommended to help improve wound care decision-making, outcomes, and reduce wound supply costs.

» G

Goal

The end that one desires to attain (Webster, 1999). In home health, a statement of what the patient wishes to attain. In contrast, an outcome is what one actually attains.

Example: A patient's spouse has a goal of independently performing the patient's dressing change before discharge from home health. Whether this goal is attained will be determined at a later point in time as the outcome.

» H

Healthcare Consultant

One who provides ethical, professional, and confidential advice to the healthcare industry for at least 1000 hours per year (American Association of Healthcare Consultants, Communication, 2007).

Health Coaching

Health coaching is a method used to enhance patient self-management. It is the practice of health education and health promotion within a coaching context, to enhance the well-being of persons and to facilitate the achievement of their health-related goals (Palmer, 2003). Health coaching assists the individual by helping him/her to reveal the change behavior needed and to overcome the ambivalence to change(s) needed. Its roots began in psychiatry in treating addicted persons.

HMO (Health Maintenance Organization)

An entity that provides, offers, or arranges for coverage of designated health services needed by members for a fixed, prepaid premium. There are three basic models of HMOs: group model, independent practice association (IPA), and staff model (USDHHS, "Office of the").

Home Care-Acquired Infection

An infection that develops 48 hours after the time of admission to home care and there was no evidence that the infection was present on admission (unless the infection was related to a previous admission to home care), and occurs at a site that home care staff could have directly contributed to its cause (McGoldrick, 2007).

Home Health Compare

A tool provided by CMS on the internet that gives consumers (in consumer's terms) home health outcomes information to help them make better informed choices about selecting a home health agency for services (USDHHS, n.d.). The following describes information given to consumers by CMS:

- The list of Home Health Agencies generated by search criteria is based on the places where they have provided services in the past.
- The services that an agency has available in these areas can change in the future. Contact the Home Health Agency to find out if it still provides the same services in your area.
- Newly Medicare-certified home health agencies may not appear in Home Health Compare for one year.
- Only Medicare-certified home health agencies are required to submit information about home health agencies.
- Agencies that exclusively serve children, or private pay, or privately insured patients are not listed here.

Home Health Agency, Types

- Hospital-based: Agency is an operating unit or department of the hospital
- Private, Not-for-Profit: Freestanding and privately developed, governed and owned non-profit
- Proprietary: Free-standing, for-profit agency
- Public: Government operated agency by a state, county, city or other unit of local government
- VNA: Visiting Nurse Associations are freestanding, voluntary, non-profit agencies governed by a board of directors and usually financed by tax-deductible contributions and earnings

Home Health Quality Initiative
In 2004-05, a private non-profit organization, the National Quality Forum (NQF), convened technical experts who endorsed measures for use in public reporting. The ten measures CMS includes in Home Health Compare (as of September 2005) reflect those recommendations. The measures (all collected via the OASIS data set) are:

- Improvement in Ambulation/Locomotion
- Improvement in Bathing
- Improvement in Transferring
- Improvement in Management of Oral Medications
- Improvement in Pain Interfering with Activity
- Acute Care Hospitalization
- Emergent Care
- Discharge to Community
- Improvement in Dyspnea
- Improvement in Urinary Incontinence

Home Health Resource Group (HHRG)
The payments for Home Health Prospective Payment System claims are based on specific payment groups, also known as Home Health Resource Groups (HHRGs) and are derived from beneficiary assessment data reported by home health agencies on the Outcome and Assessment Information Set (OASIS). The assessment items generate a clinical, functional and service "score" for a single HHRG.

Each HHRG has an associated case weight value that increases or decreases Medicare's payment for an episode of care. The HHRG is reported to Medicare using the health insurance PPS (HIPPS) code set (Medicare Payment Advisory Commission, "Home health care", 2006).

» I

Incidence
The number of new cases of a specific disease occurring during a certain period in a population at risk (Dorland's, 2000).

Example: The number of new cases of Diabetes in children within a certain year.

Independent Practice Association (IPA)
A legal entity organized and directed by physicians in private practice to negotiate contracts with insurance companies on their behalf. The IPA negotiates contracts with insurers, credentials and inspects member physicians, disperses payment to physicians, conducts utilization review and quality assurance, and insures fiscal integrity of the IPA itself (Independent Practice Associations, n.d.)

Institute of Medicine of the National Academies (Often referred to as the IOM). A federally funded agency that serves as an advisor to the federal government about matters of biomedical science, medicine and health (Institute of Medicine, n.d.). The IOM released *Crossing the Quality Chasm, A New Health System for the 21st Century,* the eye-opening report that revealed that health care in America was often found to be harmful, often failing to deliver its potential benefits, while frustrating patients and clinicians (Institute of Medicine, "About").

» J

Joint Commission on Accreditation of Healthcare Organizations, The
A private, not-for-profit organization that accredits hospitals, home health agencies and other healthcare providers according to pre-established standards. Healthcare providers volunteer to go through the accreditation process and pay for this service (Joint Commission on Accreditation of Healthcare Organizations, 2006).

» L

Leap Frog Group
The Leap Frog Group officially launched in Nov. 2000 is a voluntary program aimed at mobilizing employer purchasing power of healthcare. The founders realized that they could take "leaps" forward with their employees, retirees and families by rewarding hospitals that implement significant improvements in quality and safety (Leap Frog Group).

Length of Service
Date of home health start of care through date of home health discharge. The length of service is typically stated as the number of 60-day episodes for which care was provided from the start of care.

Example: The home health patient was on service or had a length of stay of 1.3 episodes of care.

Low Utilization Payment Adjustment (LUPA)
A per visit payment established by Medicare for patients who are discharged from home care services with four or less visits. LUPA rates for a home health agency are generally reported internally as a percentage.

» M

Managed Care
Health care systems that integrate the financing and delivery of appropriate health care services to covered individuals by arrangements with selected providers to furnish a comprehensive set of health care services, standards for selection of the care providers, quality assurance programs, utilization review, and significant financial incentives associated with the plan. Managed care is a synonym for PPO (Preferred Provider Organization), HMO (Health Maintenance Organization), MCO (Managed Care Organization), and POS (Point of Service) (Huntington, 1997).

Examples: Aetna, Inc., Humana, Inc., Wellpoint, Inc., CIGNA, Kaiser Permanente

Access webiste for further information: http://insurance.freeadvice.com/insurance_help.php/108_123_152.htm

Managed Care Plans
Health insurance plans intended to reduce unnecessary health care costs through a variety of mechanisms. The programs may be provided in a variety of settings, such as a Health Maintenance Organization (HMO), Independent Practice Association (IPA), Preferred Provider Organization (PPO), and the like (Huntington, 1997). These mechanisms include:

- Economic incentives for physicians and patients to select less costly forms of care
- Programs for reviewing the medical necessity of specific services
- Increased beneficiary cost sharing
- Controls on inpatient admissions and lengths of stay
- The establishment of cost-sharing incentives for outpatient surgery
- Selective contracting with health care providers
- Intensive management of high-cost health care cases

Medicaid
State public assistance programs that are provided to eligible persons, regardless of age, who have insufficient income to pay for healthcare. Women and children comprise Medicaid's primary recipients (Huntington, 1997).

Medicare Advantage Plan
A Medicare program that gives beneficiaries more choices among health plans. Everyone who has Medicare Parts A and B is eligible, except those who have End-Stage Renal Disease (unless certain exceptions apply). Medicare Advantage Plans were once called Medicare + Choice Plans (USDHHS,"Glossary").

Medicare Certified
A healthcare provider that meets the Centers for Medicare and Medicaid Services (CMS) conditions of participation (Ferris, 2006).

Medicare Prescription Drug, Improvement, and Modernization Act of 2003
Provision of prescription drugs under Part D for Medicare beneficiaries.

Medicare Modernization Updates can be located at:
http://www.cms.hhs.gov/MMAUpdate/

MedPAC (Medicare Payment Advisory Commission)
An independent federal body established by the Balanced Budget Act of 1997 to advise the US Congress on issues affecting Medicare Programs. MedPAC also advises regarding access to care, quality of care, and other issues affecting Medicare. MedPAC issues two reports in March and June of each year entitled Report to Congress (Medicare Payment Advisory Commission, 2005).

MedQIC (Medicare Quality Improvement Community)
A national knowledge forum for healthcare and quality improvement professionals sponsored by CMS to support and promote its Medicare Quality Improvement Program and its contractors, the QIOs, to help Medicare providers deliver the right care to every Medicare beneficiary, every time (Medicare Quality Improvement Community). The information found on its website includes interventions, tools, resources, literature and success stories.

Access more information about the Medicare Quality Improvement Community via website: http://www.medqic.org

Moist Wound Healing
Providing an environment for the wound bed that retains moisture, resulting in enhanced healing, less pain, reduced risk of infection, fewer dressing changes, and reduced cost. Moist wound healing achieves better outcomes than wet-to-dry gauze dressings (van Rijswijk, 2004).

» N

National Provider Identifier (NPI)
A 10 digit, intelligence-free numeric identifier required by HIPAA for each healthcare provider. Intelligence-free means that this number does not carry information about the healthcare provider, e.g., state located in, provider type or specialization (USDHHS, "NPI fact", 2006).

Nosocomial Infection
An infection originating in a hospital when a patient received care in an acute care setting prior to receiving care in the home and the infection was identified within the first 48 hours of being admitted to the home care organization; or the infection at a surgical site was identified within the first 30 days from the date of surgery if no implant is left in place; or the infection develops within one year from the date of a surgical implantation of a permanent nonhuman-derived foreign body and the infection does not appear to be related to the operative procedure and the infection involves any part of the body that was opened or manipulated during surgery (Rhinehart and McGoldrick, 2007).

» O

OASIS (Outcome and ASsessment Information Set)
Data items required by CMS that are assessed upon patient admission and at other time points during the home health length of stay that generate agency reimbursement and patient outcomes.

Outcome
The way something turns out; a result, a consequence. A homecare outcome is not a process, nor a care plan, nor a goal. It's often the result of care rendered (Huffman, 2005b).

Example: A goal is what you desire to achieve; an outcome is what is achieved. Goals are listed on the CMS 485 (also known as the home health plan of care). Standardized home health outcomes are generated, measured, and risk-adjusted through the OASIS instrument.

CMS defines a home health outcome as a change in patient health status between two or more points in time that may be due to the care provided and/or the natural progression of the illness. OASIS outcomes are used in home health Outcome-Based Quality Improvement (OBQI) and Outcome-Based Quality Monitoring (OBQM).

Example: OASIS outcomes are divided into three primary types.

1. End-result or health status outcomes that are further subdivided into two types:
   a. Improvement outcomes
   b. Stabilization outcomes
2. Utilization outcomes
   a. Acute care hospitalization
   b. Emergent care
   c. Discharge disposition

End-result and Utilization outcomes appear in the OBQI Risk-Adjusted and Descriptive Outcomes Report. These are further delineated as follows:

Risk-Adjusted Outcomes

- Improvement in Grooming
- Stabilization in Grooming
- Improvement in Upper Body Dressing
- Improvement in Lower Body Dressing
- Improvement in Bathing
- Stabilization in Bathing
- Improvement in Toileting
- Improvement in Transferring
- Stabilization in Transferring
- Improvement in Ambulation/Locomotion
- Improvement in Eating
- Improvement in Light Meal Preparation
- Stabilization in Light Meal Preparation
- Improvement in Laundry
- Stabilization in Laundry
- Improvement in Housekeeping
- Stabilization in Housekeeping
- Improvement in Shopping
- Stabilization in Shopping
- Improvement in Phone Use
- Stabilization in Phone Use
- Improvement in Management of Oral Medications
- Improvement in Dyspnea
- Improvement in Urinary Tract Infection
- Improvement in Urinary Incontinence
- Improvement in Bowel Incontinence
- Improvement in Confusion Frequency
- Discharged to Community
- Acute Care Hospitalization
- Any Emergent Care Provided

Descriptive Outcomes (Not yet Risk-adjusted)

- Stabilization in Management of Oral Medications
- Improvement in Speech and Language
- Stabilization in Speech and Language
- Improvement in Pain Interfering with Activity
- Improvement in Number of Surgical Wounds
- Improvement in Status of Surgical Wounds
- Improvement in Cognitive Functioning
- Stabilization in Cognitive Functioning
- Improvement in Anxiety Level
- Stabilization in Anxiety Level
- Improvement in Behavior Problem Frequency

Adverse Event Outcomes
See definition for: Adverse Event Outcome

Outcomes Aggregation
To tally the outcomes for a distinct patient group. Aggregated outcomes can be reported as a percentage, or as a percentage of patients who have met or who have not met an outcome. A percentage can also be calculated for those whom the outcome is not applicable.

Example: OASIS outcomes are aggregated into a whole or a single percentage at the national level and the agency's own prior level to give agencies a benchmark by which to compare their own outcome results.

Outcome-Based Quality Improvement (OBQI)
A systematic approach implemented by homecare agencies to continuously improve the quality of care provided. The OASIS instrument used by homecare clinicians for admission, follow-up, resumption of care, transfer, and discharge generates the patient's outcomes used in OBQI.
Access website: http://www.cms.hhs.gov/HomeHealthQualityInits/16_HHQIOASISOBQI.asp

Outcome-Based Marketing
The use of clinical and financial outcomes to market home health products and services.

Example: Home Health Compare outcomes can be reflected in graph form and used to market an agency's quality and services.

Outcome Indicator (See Outcome Measure, Health)

Outcomes Integration
The process of incorporating clinical, financial and satisfaction outcomes into agency operations, quality improvement, business strategy and marketing plans.

Outcome Measure, Health
An indicator or parameter that is assessed or evaluated to reflect the result due to a clinical intervention (Blancett & Flarey, 1998).

Example:
1. Emergent care due to fall or injury
2. Patient independently demonstrates use of blood glucometer by discharge

Outcome Measurement
The process of observing, describing, and quantifying outcome indicators (Blancett and Flarey, 1998).

Example: The registered physical therapist determines the patient's functional independence measure (FIM™ Instrument) scores at discharge. The therapist is assessing one of the patient's outcome measures.

Outcome Report
A written summary of outcome results that have been measured over a period of time.

Example: The following outcome reports are available to home health agencies:
1. Risk-adjusted and Descriptive Outcomes Report
2. Adverse Event Outcomes Report

Outcome, Process, and Structure Quality Measures
(National Quality Measures Clearinghouse)

Outcome of care: An outcome of care is a health state of a patient resulting from health care.
Process of care: A process of care is a health care service provided to, on behalf of, or by a patient appropriately based on scientific evidence of efficacy or effectiveness.
Structure of care: Structure of care is a feature of a healthcare organization or clinician relevant to its capacity to provide health care.
Access website: http://www.qualitymeasures.ahrq.gov/contact/coninclusion.aspx

Outlier
Additional payment that is made to the 60-day case-mix episode payment for beneficiaries who incur unusually large costs. The amount of the outlier payment is a proportion of the amount of imputed costs beyond the threshold amount for each case mix group (USDHHS, "PPS Overview").

» P

Patient Safety Goals, National
National Patient Safety Goals were established by The Joint Commission to promote specific improvements in patient safety (Joint Commission on Accreditation of Healthcare Organizations).

Example: Patient safety goals include areas of patient identification, communication, safety of medications, health care-associated infections, reconciliation of medications, reduction in patient falls, and patient involvement in communicating safety concerns.

Patient Satisfaction
A patient's or caregiver's level of contentment with services provided, usually reported in percentages.

Patient Population
The aggregate or totality of all patients that conform to a set of specifications (DMAA, 2004).

Example: A patient population in home health may be all patients with a primary diagnosis of congestive heart failure, all patients over 65 yrs old who are identified as a fall risk upon admission, or pediatric patients < 18 yrs of age with a primary diagnosis of asthma.

Patient Self-Management
Term used to imply the responsibility that a patient assumes for his/her own health and wellness to help prevent unnecessary exacerbations and use of acute care hospitalization. Health coaching is a new and exciting technique for home health providers to use in improving patient self-management (Huffman, 2007).

Pay-for-performance (P4P)
(See Section 1: Pay for Performance Primer.)

Physician Practice Pattern
Interventions and general response tendencies of physicians based on evidence, published data, experience and/or authority (Green, Gorenflo, and Wyszewianski, 2002).

Example: One physician may order evidence-based moist wound treatment, while another may order wet-to-dry gauze dressings.

Point-of-Care
Generally used to indicate the point at which the patient receives care from the clinician. Point-of-care may occur at the patient's place of residence, the bedside, the outpatient clinic, and the like. Also used to refer to hardware (point-of-care device) that is used by the clinician to document interventions rendered at the "point-of-care".

PPO (Preferred Provider Organization)
An arrangement where a third-party payer contracts with a group of "preferred" medical providers who furnish services at lower than usual fees in turn for prompt payment and access to a certain volume of patients (Huntington, 1997).

Predictive Modeling
A process of forecasting future health care expenditures, resource utilization, or adverse clinical events based on differences in an individual's health status. Predictive modeling is used to allocate disease management resources to the group predicted to incur high health care expenses (DMAA, 2004).

PRO (Peer Review Organization)
An organization established by the Tax Equity and Fiscal Responsibility Act of 1982 (TEFRA) to review quality of care and appropriateness of admissions, readmissions and discharges for Medicare and Medicaid. (USDHHS, "Glossary").

PPS (Prospective Payment System)
Payment for healthcare services based on information gathered at the time of admission.

Prevalence
Proportion of people in the entire population who have a disease at a certain point in time without regard to when they first got the disease (Dorland's Illustrated Dictionary, 2000).

Example: A home health wound prevalence study includes all patients with all wound types at a certain point in time.

» Q

Quality Culture (See Culture.)

Quality Improvement Organization (QIO)
Another part of the CMS quality initiative, QIOs are private organizations contracted by CMS to work with consumers, physicians, hospitals, nursing homes, and home health agencies to refine care delivery systems to make sure patients get the right care at the right time, particularly patients from underserved populations.

QIOs contract to provide their services free of charge to the consumers and providers. The QIO Program consists of 53 QIOs, responsible for each U.S. state, territory, and the District of Columbia. QIOs also safeguard the integrity of the Medicare Trust Fund by ensuring that payment is made only for medically necessary services, and investigates beneficiary complaints about quality of care (USDHHS, "Resources for").

Quality Measure(s)
The degree to which health care services for individuals and populations increase the likelihood of desired health outcomes and are consistent with current professional knowledge (National Institutes of Health, "Quality Measures,").

Example: There are hospital, home health, nursing home and physician quality measures. See Section 1: Pay for Performance Primer.

Quality of Life Measure
Refers to health-related quality of life based on those aspects of a person's overall well-being that are affected by health status or health care (Gold, 1996).

Example: Patient satisfaction surveys that address well-being are sometimes referred to as a quality of life measure.

Quality of Care
The degree to which health care services for individuals and populations increase the likelihood of desired health outcomes and are consistent with current professional knowledge (Institute of Medicine, 2001).

Query, Queries
An inquiry.

Example: The term query is often used in home care when one is filtering information through software to obtain more specific data. Instructions for the use of the OBQI Outcome Tally Report suggest the use of queries to "drill-down" to more specific data needed to conduct an investigation of a target outcome.

» R

Random Sampling
Selection of subjects for study that ensures that every subject has an equal chance of being selected (Polit, Beck and Hungler, 2001). Home Health agencies use random sampling when selecting medical records for performance improvement.

Example: Tossing a coin to select subjects is a simple example of random sampling.

Rate
A score derived by dividing the number of cases that meet a criterion for quality (the numerator) by the number of eligible cases within a given time frame (the denominator), where the numerator cases are a subset of the denominator cases.

Example: Number of patients with Diabetes Mellitus who had a HbA1c performed within the last 12 months divided by the total number of patients with Diabetes Mellitus in the same time period.

Recertification
The process of reviewing a homecare patient's plan of care to determine if homecare services need to be continued for an additional 60-day episode.

Reimbursement, PPS
An agency's prospective payment system (PPS) payment for a 60-day episode of care. Reimbursement = PPS payment amount (x) patient's case mix adjustment (x) the agency's area wage index.

Reliability
The consistency with which an instrument measures an attribute. An outcome measure is considered reliable if it is consistently reproducible (Polit, Beck and Hungler, 2001).

Example: A scale that measures your weight is reliable if it displays the same number of pounds when you weigh yourself each time, provided you have not gained or lost weight.

Resource Utilization
The means drawn upon to deliver a service, typically described as human, financial, technological, mechanical, and so forth.

Example: Resource utilization in homecare includes numbers of staff to conduct visits and numbers and types of supplies used during care.

Return on Investment (ROI)
A metric used to assess, report, and compare the value of intervention programs or equipment use.

Risk-Adjusted and Descriptive Outcome Report
An OBQI outcome report that is divided into two parts. The first part contains outcomes that are risk-adjusted and the second part contains outcomes that are considered descriptive in nature. The descriptive outcomes will likely be risk-adjusted in the future (USDHHS, 2006).

Example: Home health agencies are provided with the OBQI Risk-Adjusted and Descriptive Outcome Report to review their outcomes for both a current and prior period, and compare these with a national mean.

Revenue Recovery
A method used in home health whereby a consultant reviews billing and OASIS accuracy to determine if reimbursement dollars needed to treat the patient were inadvertently unclaimed. Corrections are made to the medical record and the Request for Anticipated Payment (RAP) is resubmitted.

Risk Adjustment
A statistical approach that minimizes the possibility that differences in outcomes between comparison groups are due to factors other than the care provided by the agency (USDHHS, 2006).

Example: Patient risk factors can account for differences in patient outcomes unless they are risk-adjusted in an attempt to control this influence. Improvement in bathing, Improvement in grooming, and Improvement in ambulation are some of the risk-adjusted OASIS outcomes used in OBQI.

Risk Assessment, Home Health
A tool used by many home health providers at the Start of Care (SOC), Resumption of Care (ROC) and at Recertification to determine risk for experiencing an adverse event or developing a certain condition during a length of service.

Examples: Assessments often inlude fall risk, pressure ulcer risk, (e.g., Braden and Norton Scales), acute care hospitalization risk, and emergent care risk.

» S

Standard of Care
An intervention that is generally implemented for all patients with the problem for which the standard applies (Humphrey and Milone-Nuzzo, 1996).

Example: An agency adopts the use of the American Diabetes Association guidelines to provide care for all patients with a primary or secondary diagnosis of Diabetes Mellitus. This becomes an agency standard of care.

Statistical Significance
Results not likely due to chance (Polit, Beck and Hungler, 2001). OBQI outcome reports have statistical significance provided. Significance is one factor that helps an agency select a target outcome for improvement or reinforcement.

Example: For the outcome, Improvement in Ambulation, a significance level of 0.08 denotes a probability > 90% that the difference between the agency's results and the source sample is real. OBQI recommends that agencies select outcomes with significance less than or equal to .10 to consider as target outcomes.

Strategic Collaboration
A working relationship among referral sources, healthcare providers, and/or supply vendors where data, experiences, and research is shared to achieve an improvement in joint outcomes.

Example: An agency enters a strategic collaborative relationship with its local hospital whereby the hospital shares its most common discharge diagnoses, percentage of patients admitted for home care, and its readmission rate for patients with CHF. The agency in turn shares its OASIS outcomes of acute care hospitalization and disease management outcomes. They strategize how to improve the outcomes and reduce the acute care hospitalization of this patient group.

Supply Costs per Diagnosis
Average home health supply costs used in a 60-day episode by diagnosis.

Example: Wound supply costs include the dressing, cleansing agent(s), debriding agent, gloves, syringes, drape, disposal, etc. Some agencies calculate the specific costs, and some have a percentage of charges that is allocated to the cost of supplies.

Supply Utilization
Supplies used; also sometimes referred to as cost of supplies.

» T

Target Outcome
An OASIS outcome selected through the model of OBQI for remediation or reinforcement by the agency (USDHHS, 2006).

Example: An agency uses the OBQI model or framework to select their target outcome for further investigation and study.

Outcome Tally Report
There are two OBQI Tally Reports: Case Mix Tally Report and the Outcome Tally Report. These are used by agencies to select patients for investigation and medical record review after a target outcome has been selected for study (Huffman, 2005).

Trending
Looking at attributes or occurrences of a patient population over time (Polit, Beck, and Hungler, 2001).

Example: An agency looks at patient falls or wound infections from month-to-month or quarter-to-quarter to determine if a trend in these adverse events is occurring. This review determines if the incidence of infection or trend is improving or worsening over time.

» U

URAC
Utilization Review Accreditation Committee, also known as the American Accreditation Healthcare Commission. URAC is the largest accrediting body for healthcare that accredits any organization that meets standards including hospitals, HMOs, PPOs, and other provider groups (URAC, 2006).

Usual care
Patient interventions that vary from one physician or clinician to the other (Tinetti, et al., 2002) and are determined by education, experience and expertise.

Example: A patient has a diagnosis of hypertension and has a physician's order for blood pressure (BP) every visit. During the home visit, some nurses take the BP while the patient is seated. Some take the blood pressure while the patient is lying down. Some take the BP while patient is seated and lying down. Each clinician decides how the blood pressure will be taken during the home visit.

Utilization Outcome (See OASIS outcome)

Utilization Review (UR)
A mechanism used by some insurers and employers to evaluate health care rendered for appropriateness, necessity, and quality. Some hospitals also have a UR committee or team that reviews medical records for appropriateness of care (Huntington, 1997).

»V

Validity

The degree to which an instrument measures what it is supposed to measure (Polit, Beck and Hungler, 2001).

Example: There are different types of validity, such as content validity, where experts analyze an instrument's content to determine if the instrument adequately covers the subject area being measured. In home health, different tools are used to measure patient's responses or assessment. These tools must be considered valid to be worthy of use. Some examples are the OASIS instrument and wound risk assessment tools.

Value-Based Purchasing

The Agency for Health care Research and Quality (AHRQ, "Theory and Reality") states that the concept of value-based health care purchasing is that buyers should hold providers of health care accountable for both cost and quality of care. Value-based purchasing brings together information on the quality of health care, including patient outcomes and health status, with data on the dollar outlays going towards health. It focuses on managing the use of the health care system to reduce inappropriate care and to identify and reward the best-performing providers. This strategy can be contrasted with more limited efforts to negotiate price discounts, which reduce costs, but do little to ensure that quality of care is improved.

The key elements of value-based purchasing include:

- Contracts spelling out the responsibilities of employers as purchasers with selected insurance, managed care, and hospital and physician groups as suppliers.
- Information to support the management of purchasing activities.
- Quality management to drive continuous improvements in the process of health care purchasing and in the delivery of health care services.
- Incentives to encourage and reward desired practices by providers and consumers.
- Education to help employees become better heath care consumers.

Variance
A state or quality varying or changing from the standard (Agnes, 2003).

Example: A care pathway is formulated to guide the clinician to deliver prescribed interventions over a defined period of time. If the patient is discharged earlier or later than the anticipated time, the patient is said to have a variance. A variance can be positive or negative. Some variances for home health include financial, lives alone, and difficulty reading/writing.

Variance management
The identification of causes of variance from planned length of stay or service, and the action taken to minimize or eliminate its effect on patient progress (Hill, 1999).

Example: An agency captures the variance of "financial difficulty" as it studies its patient outcomes related to compliance with diabetes standards of care. It is noted that this variance occurs 68% of the time for patients living in a particular geographic area. Having recognized this, the agency attempts to decrease this variance for this patient group by having increased involvement of social work services in this locale.

Visits by Discipline
The number of visits made by each discipline in a 60-day episode of care (Huffman, 2005b).

Example: Agency executives must know the number of visits that agency staff make to manage specific diagnoses effectively. This is a critical factor in determining overall costs of care.

» W

Wound care outcomes
Results of wound care that are divided broadly into three categories:
1. Clinical efficacy
2. Health-related quality of life
3. Health economics (Soon and Chen, 2004).

Examples:
1. Clinical efficacy: Percent of wounds healed, change in wound dimensions, wound infection rate.
2. Health related quality of life: Perceived pain, anxiety or fear; physical ability to carry out activities, experience with symptoms.
3. Health economics: Direct costs to include dressings, cleansing agents, disposal, visit costs to include mileage.

Subsection B
Technology

Data Mining
The computerized extraction of implicit, previously unknown, and potentially useful information from large data sets or databases. Data mining is an umbrella term usually associated with extracting clinical and financial data to identify trends.

Example: Data mining capability is typically purchased or accessed as a paid subscription by home health providers to extract meaningful data not readily available through OBQI outcome reports.

Digital Imagery
The process of taking digital images (pictures) for use in patient care management. In home health, digital imagery is most often used for wound care. Digital cameras are being used because of their high resolution capability. Wireless applications through cameras and cell phones are also used.

Electronic Data Interchange (EDI)
The transfer of data between different companies using networks, such as value added networks or the Internet (EDI).

Hardware
The computer and its equipment collaterals, such as the mouse, keyboard, monitor, and printer.

Micro Diagnostics
The use of small devices for recording diagnostic data. For example, a wristwatch-type device is available for recording EKG.

Patient Encounter
The interactive transmission of data between the patient and the nurse/therapist where decisions can be made (Chetney, 2003).

Personal Digital Assistant (PDA)
A handheld computer for managing contacts, appointments and tasks. It typically includes a name and address database, calendar, to-do list and notes. Wireless PDAs may also offer e-mail, Web browsing and cell phone service. Data are synchronized between the PDA and desktop computer via a cabled or wireless connection (The Business Technology Network).

Scan Technology, Scanner, Scan Device

An optical device that reads a printed page or transparency and converts it into a graphics image for the computer. A scanner may "read" information and send it to another location for storage, reporting, etc. It is fairly inexpensive and can enable the user to maintain control over development of its internal documents (The Business Technology Network).

Software

The programs that run on a computer, such as Microsoft Office, Excel, Corel WordPerfect, Quicken, etc. Home health agencies also develop their own software programs for internal use.

Software Interface

A computer program format that communicates with the main operating system or communications protocol that provides a link for execution of a task.

Example: An agency needs certain financial data that its existing computer program does not generate in a meaningful or usable format. A software interface may be developed by technology staff to allow financial data to be extracted from the agency's existing database into another tool (software) and presented in a report format.

Telehealth/Telemedicine

Medical information exchanged from one site to another via electronic communication to improve a patient's health status. Telehealth and telemedicine are sometimes used interchangeably. However, telemedicine is more often associated with direct patient clinical services and telehealth is more often associated with a broader definition of remote health care (American Telemedicine Association).

Telemonitoring

The remote collection and transmission of clinical data between a patient in a distant location and a healthcare provider for the purpose of data review and response to the patient; may be automated or manual data entry (American Telemedicine Association, 2006). Telemonitoring is most often used in home health to:

1. Decrease healthcare costs
2. Alert the healthcare professional and patient that prompt action is needed to avoid decline
3. Involve the user in self-management of the patient's diagnosis or condition

According to OUTCOME*Logics*, Inc. 2006 Home Health Disease Management Readiness Survey, 32% of the 620 respondents from across the nation and D.C. use some form of telemonitoring in the care of patients with chronic conditions. Those diagnoses for which home health telemonitoring are most often used:

- CHF 98%
- Diabetes 58%
- COPD and Hypertension 57%
- Pressure Ulcer 21%

For a copy of the OUTCOME*Logics* 2006 survey results, e-mail: info@outcome-architects.com

Telephony
The science, technology, or system of communication by telephone. Telephony is gaining popularity in home health as a way to communicate with patients between scheduled in-home visits to provide more cost effective ways of providing guidance to patients and performing triage/teletriage off site (Telephony). Several companies offer telephony services to home health agencies through a central calling station or provide guidance to the agency to initiate their own patient calls.

Transtelephonic Monitoring
Monitoring that is conducted via telephonic transmission most often used to record EKG and pacemaker data. Transtelephonic monitoring gained popular use in cardiac rehabilitation by enabling someone at the base station to record and "monitor" an individual's EKG in real-time, while the person exercised in an offsite location.

Value Added Network (VAN)
A private network provider that leases communication lines to its subscribers. VANs provide specialized services such as assisting with EDI (electronic data interchange), extra security, message delivery, or access to a particular database ("Value added network").

Video Conferencing
A real-time video session between two or more users or between two or more locations.

Videophone
A telephone that is capable of both audio and video transmission.

Video Streaming
A delivery method that allows video to be transmitted live over the internet to many users/viewers simultaneously ("Video streaming").

Voice Recognition
The conversion of spoken words into computer text. Speech is first digitized and then matched against a dictionary of coded waveforms. The matches are converted into text as if the words were typed on the keyboard (PDA, 2006). Voice recognition is considered a viable way of keeping older nurses active in the workforce, who might otherwise leave practice due to inexperience with technology (Lupoli and Rizzo, 2003).

Webcast
The transmission of audio or video content over the internet. The term is derived from "web" and "broadcast". Information is transmitted only one way, which is to the listener ("Webcast").

Webconferencing
Group meetings held via the internet whereby written material is shown on the internet while simultaneously conversing about it on the telephone ("Webconferencing").

Webinar
A seminar conducted over the world wide web that is interactive between presenter and audience. It is "live" in the sense that information is presented according to an agenda with start and end time. Speaker often speaks over the telephone while presentation is shown on the monitor screen. Audiences ask questions over the phone ("Webinar").

Wireless Technology
Use of pocket personal computer (pocket PC), camera, personal digital assistant (PDA), laptop, etc., to send and receive communications, data and information without a cable or telephone line.

Subsection C
Sales & Marketing

Benefit
An asset that shows how a product can help a customer, meet a need, and/or appeal to the personal ego needs of the buyer, or to organizational or departmental needs (Rackham, 1988).

Branding
Developing and consistently communicating a set of positive characteristics that consumers can identify with and relate to the seller's name (Schenck, 2005).

Buying Influence
The role of the person who will act as a buyer for your sales objective, who will give final approval to the purchase (Rackham, 1988).

Closing
After the customer agrees to purchase, moving the customer to complete the sale. The process used by the salesperson to induce purchase of accepting the proposition (Heiman and Sanchez, 1998).

Competition
The contest between businesses for customer and sales (Rackham, 1988).

Customer
One who has purchased a product or service (Schenck, 2005). There are internal and external customers. Internal customers are those of the organization who are served by those within the same organization. External customers are those served outside the organization.

Customer Concept
What the individual feels is important to accomplish, to fix or to avoid (Heiman and Sanchez, 1998).

Feature
Facts, data, or information about your product(s) or service(s) (Rackham, 1988).

Marketing
The process by which you create and keep customers (Schenck, 2005).

Market Share
Your slice of the market pie or your portion of all the sales of products/services like yours offered in your market area (Schenck, 2005).

Positioning
Involves figuring out what meaningful and available niche in the market your business is designed to fill, filling it, and performing so well that your customers buy from you (Rackham,1988).

Prospect
One who may be interested in your product or service (Schenck, 2005).

Sales Strategy
A central, organizing statement that allows you to make a good decision about what you will do in a sales campaign or game plan (Holden, 1990).

Selling
The process between initial prospecting and the signed agreement to buy (Heiman and Sanchez, 1998).

Target Market
The market within the sphere of influence of your business (Schenck, 2005).

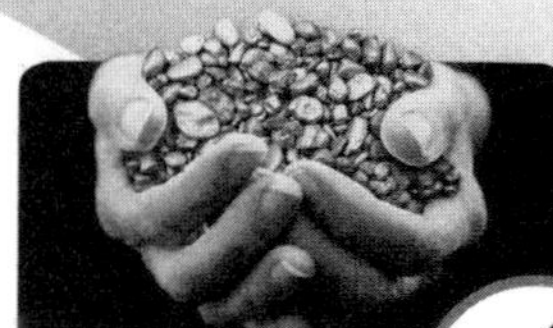

Section 4

Home Health Acronyms

AAHC	American Association for Home Care (www.aahc.org)
ADL	Activities of Daily Living
ADR	Additional Documentation Request
AHIMA	American Health Information Management Association (www.ahima.org)
AHRQ	Agency for Health Research and Quality (www.ahrq.org)
ALF	Assisted Living Facility
CASPER	Certification and Survey Provider Enhanced Program
CDC	Centers for Disease Control (www.cdc.gov)
C-F-S	Clinical-Functional-Service Domains
CHAP	Community Health Accreditation Program (www.chapinc.org)
CMS	Centers for Medicare and Medicaid Services (www.cms.gov)
CPO	Care Plan Oversight
DHHS	Department of Health and Human Services
DM	Disease Management
DMAA	Disease Management Association of America (www.dmaa.org)
DME	Durable Medical Equipment
DMO	Disease Management Organization
DRG	Diagnosis Related Group (Hospital PPS)
EBP	Evidence-based Practice
HCFA	Health Care Financing Administration
HHA	Home Health Agency/Home Health Aide
HHRG	Home Health Resource Group
HMO	Health Maintenance Organization
HIPAA	Health Insurance Portability and Accountability Act
HIPPS	Health Insurance Prospective Payment System (Codes)
IADLs	Instrumental Activities of Daily Living
ICD-CM	International Classification of Diseases-Clinical Modification
ICF	Intermediate Care Facility
IPA	Independent Practice Association
IOM	Institute of Medicine

LOS	Length of service/Length of stay
LUPA	Low utilization payment adjustment
MCO	Managed Care Organization
MedPAC	Medicare Payment Advisory Commission (www.medpac.org)
MedQIC	Medicare Quality Improvement Community (www.medqic.org)
MMA	Medicare Modernization Act (Medicare Prescription Drug, Improvement and Modernization Act of 2003)
NAHC	National Association of Home Care (www.nahc.org)
NGC	National Guidelines Clearinghouse (www.guideline.gov)
NHCPO	National Hospice and Palliative Care Organization (www.nhpco.org)
NPI	National Provider Identifier
NQMC	National Quality Measures Clearinghouse (www.qualitymeasures.ahrq.gov)
NPUAP	National Pressure Ulcer Advisory Panel (www.npuap.org)
OASIS	Outcome and ASsessment Information Set
OBRA	Omibus Budget Reconciliation Act
OIG	Office of Inspector General
OBQI	Outcome-Based Quality Improvement
OBQM	Outcome-Based Quality Monitoring
PEP	Partial Episode Payment
P4P	Pay-for-performance
POC	Point of Care/Plan of Care
PPS	Prospective Payment System
PPO	Preferred Provider Organization
PRO	Peer Review Organization
QIO	Quality Improvement Organization
QMB	Qualified Medicare Beneficiary
RAP	Request for Anticipated Payment
RHHI	Regional Home Health Intermediary
ROC	Resumption of Care
SNF	Skilled Nursing Facility
SOC	Start of Care
SSA	Social Security Administration
URAC	Utilization Review Accreditation Committee (www.urac.org)
UR	Utilization Review
VNA	Visiting Nurse Association
VNS	Visiting Nurse Service
WOCN	Wound, Ostomy and Continence Nurses Society (www.wocn.org)

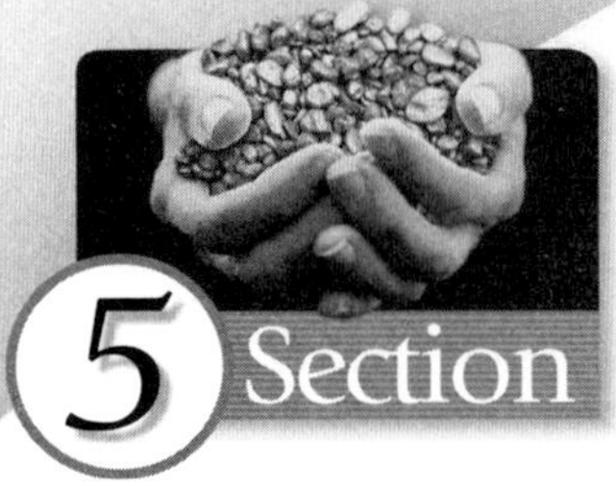

Websites for Evidence-Based Practice

This website listing is not exhaustive.

- **Agency for Healthcare Research and Quality**
  www.ahrq.gov

- **American Academy of Neurology**
  www.aan.com/professionals/practice/guidelines.cfm

- **American Academy of Pediatrics**
  www.aap.org/policy/paramtoc.html

- **American Academy of Physical Medicine and Rehabilitation**
  www.aapmr.org/hpl/pracguide/resource/htm

- **American College of Cardiology**
  www.acc.org/qualityandscience/clinical/topic/topic.htm

- **American College of Physicians**
  www.acponline.org/sci-policy/guidelines

- **American Diabetes Association**
  www.diabetes.org

- **American Heart Association**
  www.americanheart.org

- **American Lung Association**
  www.lungusa.org

- **American Psychiatric Association**
  www.psych.org/psych_pract/

- **Centers for Disease Control**
  www.cdc.gov

- **Cochrane, Collaboration, The**
  www.cochrane.org

- **Evidence-based Medicine Resources**
  www.ebmny.org/cpg.html

- **Evidence-based Nursing**
  www.ebn.bmj.com

- **National Council on Aging**
  www.ncoa.org

- **National Guideline Clearinghouse**
  www.guideline.gov

- **National Pressure Ulcer Advisory Panel**
  www.npuap.org

- **Primary Care Clinical Practice Guidelines**
  www.medicine.ucsf.edu/resources/guidelines

- **Wound, Ostomy, Continence Nurses Society**
  www.wocn.org

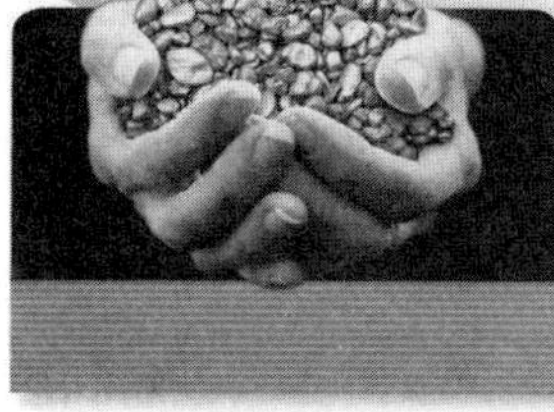

References

Agnes, M. (Ed). (2003). *Webster's New World Dictionary (4th ed.)*. NY: MacMillan.

American Management Association. Consumer driven healthcare: Wave of the future; still in its infancy. Retrieved January 16, 2007 from http://www.amanet.org/editorial/healthcare_brief.htm

American Telemedicine Association. Terminology. Retrieved February 23, 2007 from http://www.atmeda.org/ICOT/Terminology.pdf

Andersen, B. (2006, April). Promoting the value of home care in the new chronic care environment. Presentation at McKesson Horizon Homecare and Hospice Conference, Springfield, MO.

Association of Healthcare Consultants. (n.d.). Definition. Retrieved February 23, 2007 at http://www.healthcon.org.

Baker, G. et al.(2003). Pay-for-performance incentive programs in healthcare: Market dynamics and business process. Retrieved February 21, 2007 from http://www.vips.com/pdf/white%20papers/P4Pincentive_wp.pdf

Benefield, L.E. (2002). Evidence-based practice: Basic strategies for success. *Home Healthcare Nurse*, 20(12), pp.803-807.

Blancett, S. and Flarey, D. (1998). *Healthcare outcomes: collaborative, path-based approaches.* Gaithersburg, MD: Aspen.

Briggs National Quality Improvement/Hospital Reduction Study. (2006, January). Briggs Corporation: Author.

Chetney, R. (2003). Home care technology and telehealth: The future is here! *Home Healthcare Nurse*, 21(10), 645.

Contino, D. S. (2004). What's your project's ROI? Information Technology Extra. *Nursing Management*. 35(2), 39-40.

HMO. (n.d.). Definition. Retrieved February 21, 2007 from http://en.wikipedia.org/wiki/Managed_care

Disease Management Association of America. (n.d.). Definition. Retrieved February 23, 2007 from www.dmaa.org/definition.html

Disease Management Association of America. (2004). *Dictionary of Disease Management Terminology*. Washington, DC: author.

Dorland's Illustrated Medical Dictionary. (29th ed.). (2000). WB Saunders.

EDI. (n.d.). Webopedia. Retrieved January 20, 2007 at http://www.webopedia.com/TERM/E/EDI.html

Ferris, M. (2006). *Field guide to selling home care services with legendary results*. Home Care Marketing Solutions: Chapel Hill, NC.

Gitomer, J. (2006). *Jeffrey Gitomer's little black book of connections: 6.5 assets for networking your way to rich relationships*. Austin, TX: Bard Press.

Goddin, S. (2003). *Purple Cow*. New York, New York: Penguin Group.

Gold, M.R. (1996). *Cost-effectiveness in health and medicine*. New York, New York: Oxford University Press.

Green, A.C., Gorenflo, D.W. and Wyszewianski, L. (2002). Validating an instrument for selecting interventions to change physician practice patterns: A Michigan consortium for family practice research study. *Journal of Family Practice*, 51(11), p.938.

Greenburg, M.E. and Schultz, C. (2002). Telephone nursing: Client experiences and perceptions. *Nursing Economics*, 20(4),181-190.

Hagenow, N.R. (1999). Examining the dollars and cents of care. *Nursing Management*, 30 (3), 23-25.

Heiman, S. and Sanchez, D. (1998). *The new strategic selling*. Clayton South, Australia: Warner Books.

HHQI National Campaign 2007 Goal. (2007). Retrieved on January 20, 2007 from http://www.homehealthquality.org/hh/goal/default.aspx

Hill, M. (1999). Outcomes measurement requires nursing to shift to outcome-based practice. *Nursing Administration*, 24 (1), 1-9.

Holden, J. (1990). *Power-base selling*. John Wiley & Sons, Inc.

Home health pay-for-performance (2006, December 13). Abt Associates. PowerPoint Presentation. CMS Open Door Forum for Home Health. Retrieved February 21, 2007 from http://www.cms.gov/DemoProjectsEvalRpts/downloads/HHPP_Presentation.pdf

Huffman, M. (2005a). Compliance, health outcomes, and partnering in PPS: Acknowledging the patient's agenda. *Home Healthcare Nurse*, 23(1), pp.3-28.

Huffman, M. (2005b). *Implementing outcome-based homecare: A work book of obqi, care pathways and disease management.* Sudbury, MA: Jones and Bartlett Publishers.

Huffman, M. (2005c). Six financial outcomes essential to successful home health disease management. *The Remington Report*, 13 (4), 10-12.

Huffman, M. (2006a). Unlock the power of strategic collaboration across settings: It's all about outcomes! *The Remington Report*, 14(4), 36.

Huffman, M. (2006b). Home health disease management: Seizing the opportunity. OUTCOME*Logics*, Inc. White Paper. Retrieved January 15, 2007 from http://www.outcomelogics.co/whitepaper

Huffman, M. (2007, in press). Health coaching: A new and exciting technique to enhance patient self-management and improve outcomes. *Home Healthcare Nurse*.

Humphrey, C.J. and Milone-Nuzzo, P. (1996). *Orientation to home care nursing*. Gaithersburg, MD: Aspen.

Huntington, Judith A. (1997, January 6). Glossary for managed care. *Online Journal of Issues in Nursing*. Retrieved May 2, 2006 from http://www.nursingworld.org/ojin/tpc2/tpc2_gls.htm

Independent practice associations: A primer for physician assistants. (n.d.). Retrieved on February 21, 2007 from http://www.aapa.org/gandp/ipas.html

Institute of Medicine. (2001, March). Crossing the quality chasm: A new health system for the 21st century. Retrieved December 1, 2006 from http://www.nap.edu/books/0309072808/html/

Institute of Medicine. About. Retrieved February 22, 2007 from http://www.iom.edu/CMS/AboutIOM.aspx

Johnson, M., Maas, M. and Moorehead, S. (Eds.). (2000). *Iowa outcomes project: Nursing outcomes classification. 2nd Edition.* Mosby.

Joint Commission on Accreditation of Healthcare Organizations. *Comprehensive accreditation manual for home care. (2006).* Oakbrook Terrace, IL: Joint Commision Resources.

Joint Commission on Accreditation of Healthcare Organizations. (1994). *Framework for improving performance: From principles to practice.* Oakbrook Terrace, IL: Joint Commission Resources.

Joint Commission on Accreditation of Healthcare Organizations. (2007). Home care national patient safety goals. Retrieved February 23, 2007 from http://www.jointcomission.org/PatientSafety/NationalPatientSafetyGoals/07_ome_npsg.htm

Keys to successful change. (n.d.). Retrieved December 11, 2006 from http://www.robinsonleadership.com/learning/keys.php

Leap Frog Group (n.d.). How and why. Retrieved February 15, 2007 at http://www.leapfroggroup.org/about_us/how_and_why

Lupoli, J.& Rizzo,V.M., (2003). The impact of technology on the older nurse. *Home Healthcare Nurse,* 21(10), 691-692.

McGoldrick, M. (2007). *Home care infection prevention and control program.* Saint Simons Island, GA: Home Health Systems. http://www.HomeCareandHospice.com

Medicare Payment Advisory Commission (2005). About MedPAC. Retrieved February 23, 2007 from http://www.medpac.gov/about_medpac/index.cfm?section=about_medpac

Medicare Payment Advisory Commission. Home health care services payment system: Payment basics. Retrieved on November 20, 2006 from http://www.medpac.gov/publications/other_reports_/Dec05_payment_basics_HHA.pdf

Medicare Quality Improvement Community. Retrieved on February 21, 2007 from http://www.medqic.org.

Merriam-Webster's Collegiate Dictionary. (10th Ed.). (2002). Merriam-Webster, Inc.

Miller, W. & Rollnick, S. (1990). *Motivational interviewing: Preparing people for change.* New York: Guilford Press.

National Association of Home Care and Hospice. (2005, March) NAHC Report. Implementation of pay-for-performance/IT systems for home health and other providers strongly recommended by MedPAC. Washington, DC: author.

National Institutes of Health. National Heart, Lung and Blood Institute. (2004, August). Seventh report of the Joint National Committee on prevention, detection, evaluation, and treatment of high blood pressure. Retrieved February 21, 2007 from http://www.nhlbi.nih.gov/guidelines/hypertension/jnc7full.htm

National Institutes of Health. National Quality Measures Clearinghouse. Agency for Healthcare Research and Quality. (n.d.). Glossary. Retrieved February 21, 2007 from http://www.qualitymeasures.ahrq.gov/resources/glossary.aspx

Ovington, L.G. (2001). Hanging wet-to-dry dressings out to dry. *Home Healthcare Nurse,* 19(8), 477.

Palmer, S.(2003). Health coaching to facilitate the promotion of healthy behavior and achievement of health-related goals. *International Journal of Health Promotion and Education,* 41(3), 91-93.

Polit, D.F., Beck, C.T., Hungler, B.P.(2001) *Essentials of nursing research: Methods, appraisal, and utilization*. 5th Edition. Lippincott.

Quality Insights of Pennsylvania. Organizational culture in home health: Introduction. Retrieved February 22, 2007 from http://www.medqic.org/dcs/ContentServer?cid=11422803146308&pagename=Medqic%2FMQ%2FToolTemplate&c=MQTools

Rackham, N. (1988). *Spin-selling.* McGraw-Hill Inc.

Remington, L. (2006). Publisher's message. *The Remington Report,* 14 (6), 5.

Rhinehart, E., McGoldrick, M. (2006). Infection Control in Home Care and Hospice for the Association for Professionals in Infection Control and Epidemiology, Inc., (APIC). Sudbury, MA: Jones and Bartlett.

Rosenblum, B. (2006) The national telehealth value study. *The Remington Report,*14(3), Special Case Study Section.

Schenck, B.F. (2005). *Small business marketing for dummies. 2nd Edition.* Wiley Publishing.

Sheyte, R. and Struk, C. (2003). Technology tidbits: What is data decision support and why should I care? *Home Healthcare Nurse,* 21(10), 652.

Soon, S.L. and Chen, S.C. (2004, May). What are wound outcomes? *Wounds,* 16(5), pp.150-156.

The Business Technology Network. (n.d.). Tech Encyclopedia. PDA. Retrieved February 23, 2007 from http://www.techweb.com/encyclopedia/defineterm.jhtml?term=PDA

Telephony: Definition. (n.d.). Retrieved February 23, 2007 from http://encarta.msn.com/dictionary_/telephony.html

Tinetti, ME., Baker, D., Gallo, W.T., Nanda, A., Charpentier,P., & O'Leary, J. (2002). Evaluation of restorative care versus usual care for older adults receiving an acute episode of home care. *JAMA,* 287(16), 2098.

URAC. (2006). Frequently asked questions. Retrieved February 23, 2007 from http://www.urac.org/about_faqs.aspx

***Note: The following sixteen references are from the U.S. Department of Health and Human Services. (Cited in text as USDHHS)**

Agency for Healthcare Research and Quality. (n.d.). Theory and reality of value-based purchasing: Lessons from pioneers. Retrieved January 15, 2007 at www.ahrq.gov/qual/meyerrpt.htm#head1

Agency for Healthcare Research and Quality. (2002). Hospitalization in the United States. AHRQ publication no. 05-0056. Rockville, MD: author

Agency for Healthcare Research and Quality (1995). Using clinical practice guidelines to evaluate quality of care. AHCPR Publication no. 95-0045. Rockville, MD: author

Centers for Medicare and Medicaid Services, (2006). *Outcome-based quality improvement (OBQI) implementation manual.* Baltimore, MD: author

Centers for Medicare and Medicaid Services. (2006, January). NPI Fact sheet: The national provider identifier. The Medicare Learning Network: author.

Centers for Medicare and Medicaid Services. (2006, May). Home health quality initiatives: Overview. Retrieved on February 22, 2007 from http://www.cms.hhs.gov/HomeHealthQualityInits/

Centers for Medicare and Medicaid Services, (n.d.). Office of the Assistant Secretary for Planning and Evaluation (ASPE). Managed care terminology. Retrieved February 23, 2007 from http://www.aspe.hhs.gov/Progsys/Forum/mcobib.htm

Centers for Medicare and Medicaid Services. (n.d.).Glossary: Medicare advantage plan. Retrieved February 23, 2007 from http://www.medicare.gov/Glossary/ShowTerm.asp?Language=English&term=medicare+advantage+plan

Centers for Medicare and Medicaid Services. (n.d.). Home health compare. Retrieved February 23, 2007 from http://www.medicare.gov/HHCompare/Home.asp?dest=NAV/Home/About#TabTop

Centers for Medicare and Medicaid Services. (n.d.). Overview. Retrieved February 23, 2007 from http://www.cms.hhs.gov/HomeHealthQualityInits/

Centers for Medicare and Medicaid Services. (n.d.). PPS overview. Retrieved February 23, 2007 from http://www.cms.hhs.gov/HomeHealthPPS/01_Overview.asp

Centers for Medicare and Medicaid Services. (n.d.) Overview. Medicaid and SCHIP Quality Practices. Retrieved January 23, 2007 from www.cms.hhs.gov/MedicaidSCHIPQualPrac/01_Overview.asp#TopOfPage

Centers for Medicare and Medicaid Services. PVRP. Retrieved February 23, 2007 from http://www.cms.hha.gov/PVRP/01_Overview.asp

Centers for Medicare and Medicaid Services. Hospital compare quality measures. (n.d.) Retrieved February 23, 2007 from http://www.hospitalcompare.hhs.gov/Hospital/Static/AboutHospQuality.asp?dest=NAV|Home|About|QualityMeasures#TabTop

Centers for Medicare and Medicaid Services. Resources for Quality Improvement. (n.d.). Retrieved February 22, 2007 from http://www.cms.hhs.gov/QualityImprovementOrgs/01_overview.asp

Health Care Financing Administration. (2001). Quality monitoring using case mix and adverse event outcome reports: Implementing outcome based quality improvement at a home health agency. Retrieved February 23, 2007 from http://www.cms.gov/HomeHealthQualityUnits/download/HHQIOASISOBQMCaseMix.pdf

Value Added Network. (n.d.). Webopedia. Retrieved January 20, 2007 at http://www.webopedia.com/TERM/V/VAN.html

van Rijswijk, L. (2004). Moist dressings: Bridging the gap between research and practice. *Advances in Skin & Wound Care*, 17(5), 254.

Video Streaming. (n.d.). Definition. Retrieved February 8, 2007 from http://ed.wikipedia.org/streaming_med

Webster's New World College Dictionary (4th ed.). (1999). MacMillan USA.

Webcast. (n.d.). Definition. Retrieved February 8, 2007 from http://ed.wikipedia.org/wiki/webcast

Web conferencing. (n.d.). Definition. Retrieved February 8, 2007 from http://ed.wikipedia.org/wiki/web_conference

Webinar. (n.d.). Definition. Retrieved February 8, 2007 from http://ed.wikipedia.org/wiki/webinar

Notes

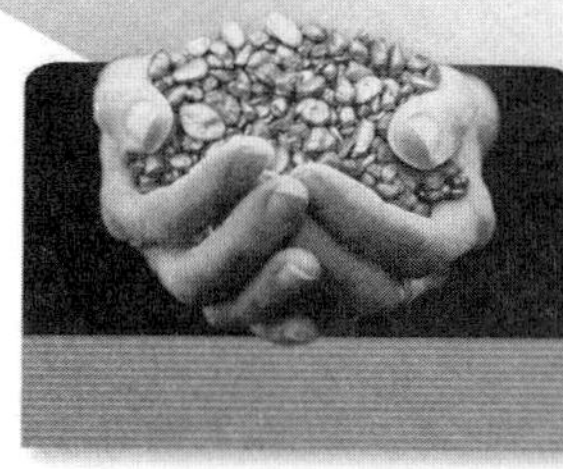

Index

Notes

Notes

Notes

Notes